# A colour atlas of
# Renal
# Diseases

## GEORGE WILLIAMS

M.D., Ph.D., F.R.C.Path.

*Reader in Pathology, University of Manchester*
*Hon. Consultant Pathologist, Manchester Royal Infirmary*

## WOLFE MEDICAL BOOKS
10 Earlham Street, London, WC2

# A COLOUR ATLAS OF RENAL DISEASES

*Copyright* © George Williams, M.D., Ph.D., F.R.C.Path. 1973
Published by Wolfe Publishing Ltd 1973
Printed by Smeets-Weert Holland
2nd Impression 1976
SBN 72340406 2

General Editor, Wolfe Medical Books
G Barry Carruthers MD (Lond)

Books in this series already published
*A colour atlas of Haematological Cytology*
*A colour atlas of General Pathology*
*A colour atlas of Oro-Facial Diseases*
*A colour atlas of Ophthalmological Diagnosis*
*A colour atlas of Renal Diseases*
*A colour atlas of Venereology*
*A colour atlas of Dermatology*
*A colour atlas of Infectious Diseases*
*A colour atlas of Ear, Nose & Throat Diagnosis*
*A colour atlas of Rheumatology*
*A colour atlas of Microbiology*
*A colour atlas of Forensic Pathology*
*A colour atlas of Paediatrics*
*A colour atlas of Histology*
*A colour atlas of General Surgical Diagnosis*
*A colour atlas of Physical Signs in General Medicine*
*A colour atlas of Tropical Medicine & Parasitology*

Some further titles now in preparation
*A colour atlas of Cardiac Pathology*
*A colour atlas of Gynaecology*
*A colour atlas of Orthopaedics*
*A colour atlas of the Liver*
*A colour atlas of Endocrinology*
*A colour atlas of Cytology*
*A colour atlas of Urology*
*A colour atlas of Staining Techniques*

# Contents

# Acknowledgements

I am indebted to my friend and colleague, Dr. James Davson, for constructive criticism of the text and for his expert advice as a nephrologist. I also wish to thank the technical staff of the University Department of Pathology for preparing the large numbers of specimens for light and electron microscopy and Mr. G. C. W. Humberstone who photographed the gross specimens.

X-ray films for Figs. 194, 195, 233 and 263 were generously provided by Dr. V. Cope; illustrations or specimens for Figs. 258–262 and 264–267 by my colleague Dr. A. R. Mainwaring; for Figs. 109, 114 and 124 by Mrs. P. A. Portch, M.Sc., and for Figs. 127, 268 and 269 by Dr. N. P. Mallick. Fig. 127 is reproduced by kind permission of Dr. George Ackerman of the Medical School, University of Arkansas. Fig. 22 was kindly provided by Dr. A. J. Barson.

Finally, may I sincerely thank Mrs. Jenni Sellar and Mrs. Jean Edwards for their patience and efficiency in typing the manuscript.

GEORGE WILLIAMS

To Mary, Paula, Gordon and "Gipsy"

# Introduction

A HEALTHY KIDNEY has a complex structure and performs many functions. Both may be significantly changed by disease which may originate in the kidney itself or involve it as complications of diseases arising in other body tissues or systems. In either case a wide variety of abnormal clinical signs and symptoms may result.

This atlas is produced from the viewpoint of a pathologist; it is therefore mainly concerned with the structural aspects of renal diseases as studied in gross specimens and microscopical preparations. To aid interpretation, appearances at both these levels have been frequently correlated. This production is directed mainly at undergraduates, who, for good reasons, often find renal diseases confusing and hard to understand—an opinion shared by not a few post-graduates as well.

Studies of structural change alone cannot provide the answers to all the problems of disease, but they are fundamental to a better understanding of them and play an important part in establishing clinical diagnosis and influencing treatment. Some of the rarer renal diseases have intentionally been omitted from this atlas, but it is hoped that the range of abnormalities illustrated is sufficiently wide to help both students and graduates understand the more common and important ones they are likely to meet.

# Presentation of Specimens

MOST ILLUSTRATIONS of gross specimens presented in this atlas incorporate a measuring scale—hence magnifications are not stated in the descriptions. Magnifications for light and electron micrographs are, however, indicated.

Many staining techniques were used in preparing the sections for histology. The three most often used in the illustrations are:

(1) a combination of haematoxylin and eosin (H and E).

(2) the periodic acid-Schiff (PAS) technique which stains basement membranes and other glyco-proteins a rose-red/magenta colour, combined with haematoxylin as a nuclear stain.

(3) the martius (yellow)-scarlet-blue (MSB) technique with which collagenous connective tissue appears blue, fibrin and muscle—red, and red blood cells—yellow.

Other useful preparations were obtained using a silver methenamine—light green (MeS) combination which gives black basement membranes against a green background, and the elastic-van Gieson (EVG) stain which colours elastic tissue blue/black, collagen red, and muscle, yellow.

Preparations in which particular components are demonstrated (e.g. amyloid with Congo Red) are individually indicated.

# Aspects of normal kidney structure

Kidney lobes

Cortex, columns of Bertin and medulla

The nephron

Renal corpuscle

Renal tubule

Macula densa

Renal lobules
Collecting tubules and ducts

Pelvic calyx
Renal papilla

EACH ADULT kidney weighs about 150 gm. and is formed of upwards of 12 lobes fused into a single organ within a fibrous capsule. Each lobe consists of an outer cortex with an underlying medulla shaped as a pyramid with its apex pointing inwards towards the pelvis; inward extensions of the cortex between the pyramids are called the columns of Bertin. Both cortex and medulla are composed of the kidney's functional units or nephrons (at least 1 million per kidney) along with their supporting connective tissues, arteries, veins, nerves and lymph vessels. Each nephron is made up of a renal corpuscle and a tubule about 5 cm. long. The corpuscle consists of a vascular capillary tuft or glomerulus enclosed within an epithelial-lined capsule (of Bowman). The latter represents the blind end of the tubular component, which, on account of its changing outline, is described as having a proximal convolution or coil followed by a loop (of Henle) with descending and ascending limbs, and a distal convolution which contacts its corpuscle of origin at a point called the macula densa. The distal convolution, which marks the extremity of the nephron, then joins a collecting tubule, the latter representing the common urinary drainage pathway of several nephrons. Such groups of nephrons together form smaller units of kidney structure called lobules which have no recognisable anatomical boundaries. Fusion of collecting tubules near the medullary apex produces larger collecting ducts which deliver the final urinary product into the pelvic calyces through small openings in the medullary papillae.

Most of the kidney cortex is made up of the renal corpuscles surrounded by the proximal and distal convoluted portions of the tubules. The medulla consists mainly of the tubular loops of Henle, collecting tubules and ducts and their vessels of blood supply. Where these two zones meet, along the base of each pyramid, a series of "streaks" or medullary rays run out for a short distance into the cortex and represent short parallel lengths of collecting tubules.

## Kidney blood supply
This is delivered by the renal artery entering the renal sinus; thereafter, by progressive division it gives rise to smaller lobar, arcuate, then interlobular branches which penetrate between the cortical renal lobules. From each interlobular artery arise several afferent arterioles, each of which supplies a glomerulus. The post-glomerular or efferent arterioles then divide into a meshwork of capillaries to supply the renal tubules between which they run. Those related to juxtamedullary glomeruli follow the course of kidney tubular loops for varying distances into the medulla as the vasa recta, forming the main blood supply to the renal papillae before looping back to join the venous drainage system at the cortico-medullary junction. Progressively larger venous tributaries carry the blood back to the renal vein which leaves the kidney through the renal sinus, usually just in front of the renal artery.

## The glomerulus
Each glomerulus consists of thin walled capillary loops which project into the space outlined by Bowman's capsule. They are arranged in groups as lobules with a supporting connective tissue core or mesangium. The wall of each capillary consists of a basement membrane lined by endothelial cells and covered externally by epithelial cells which contact the outer surface through delicate foot processes or pedicels. Within the supporting mesangium lie the mesangial or axial cells surrounded by matrix. The urinary filtrate passing from the blood plasma in the capillary lumen across the capillary wall enters the space of Bowman's capsule and thence into a renal tubule.

Medullary rays

Afferent and
efferent
arterioles

Vasa recta

Mesangium
Endothelial and
epithelial cells
Foot processes

Mesangial or
axial cells

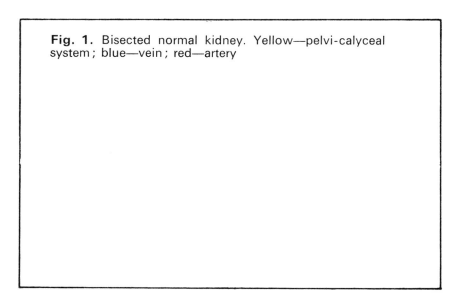

**Fig. 1.** Bisected normal kidney. Yellow—pelvi-calyceal system; blue—vein; red—artery

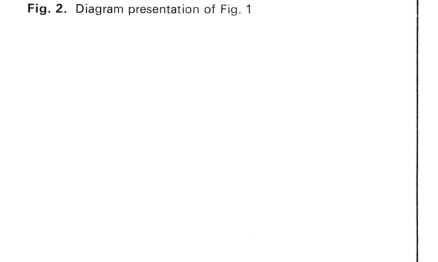

**Fig. 2.** Diagram presentation of Fig. 1

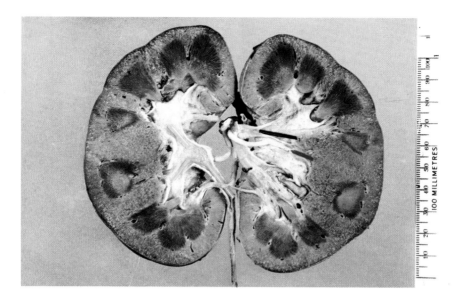

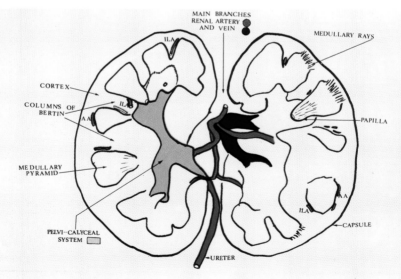

MAIN BRANCHES
RENAL ARTERY
AND VEIN

MEDULLARY RAYS

ILA

CORTEX

COLUMNS OF
BERTIN

ILA

A A

PAPILLA

MEDULLARY
PYRAMID

PELVI-CALYCEAL
SYSTEM

A A

ILA

CAPSULE

URETER

**Fig. 3.** Renal arterial supply (red) and pelvi-calyceal system (yellow) in resin cast of left kidney

**Fig. 4.** Renal arterial supply (red) ; venous drainage (blue) and pelvi-calyceal system (yellow) in resin cast of left kidney

**Fig. 5.** Diagram of juxtamedullary nephron and blood supply, showing :

aa—afferent arteriole
ea—efferent arteriole
pct—proximal convoluted tubule
dl—descending limb of Henle
al—ascending limb of Henle
dct—distal convoluted tubule
gc—glomerular corpuscle
loH—loop of Henle
vr—vasa recta

**Fig. 6.** Glomeruli, afferent arterioles and interlobular artery (MSB x 66)

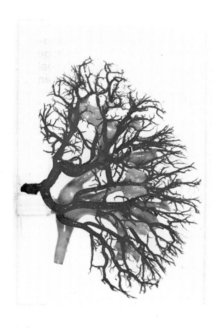

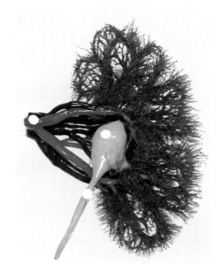

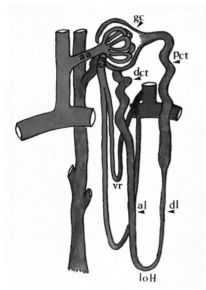

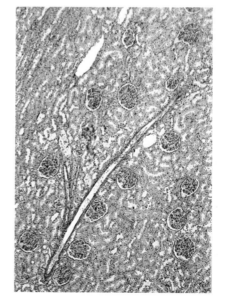

**Fig. 7.** Normal glomerular corpuscle and proximal tubules (*upper left*) (PAS x 352)

**Fig. 8.** Part of glomerular tuft, Bowman's capsule with lining epithelium and proximal tubules. Relationships of capillary basement membranes, mesangial cells (dark cytoplasm), endothelial cells and (paler) epithelial cells are shown (PAS x 1430)

**Fig. 9.** Diagram of glomerular capillary fine structure, showing:

1—capillary lumen      5—foot processes
2—epithelial cell      6—endothelial cell
3—basement membrane    7—mesangial matrix
4—red blood cell       8—mesangial cell

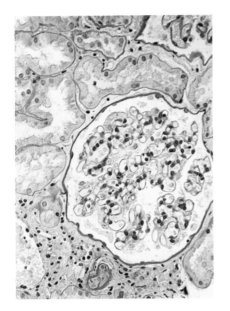
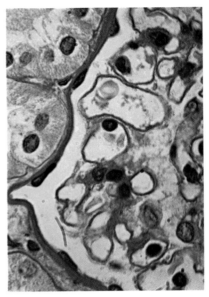
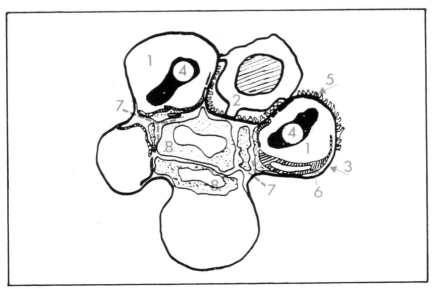

**Fig. 10.** Electron micrograph of mouse glomerulus showing features outlined in Fig. 9 (x 9000 nm)

1—capillary lumen   5—foot processes
2—epithelial cell   6—endothelial cell
3—basement membrane   7—mesangial matrix
4—red blood cell   8—mesangial cell

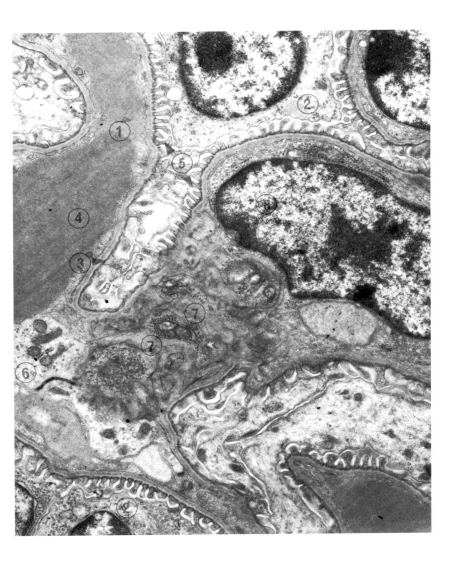

**Fig. 11.** Human glomerulus: the juxtaglomerular apparatus (JGA) at the vascular pole (6–7 o'clock) consists of modified smooth muscle cells in the wall of the afferent arteriole. In man they contain few specific granules and variable non-specific granules. Immediately below lie the modified epithelial cells of the macula densa (PAS x 330)

**Fig. 12.** Human kidney; normal proximal tubules (*below*) and distal tubule (*above*) (MSB x 1430)

**Fig. 13.** Collecting ducts and interduct capillaries (H and E x 480)

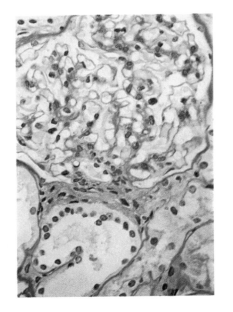

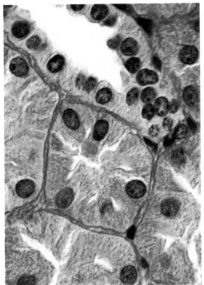

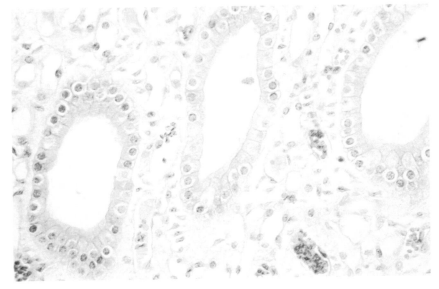

**Fig. 14.** Proximal tubule of mouse kidney, showing:

2—epithelial cell
3—basement membrane
9—mitochondria
10—microvilli
11—lysosomes
12—intertubular capillary
(x 1200 nm)

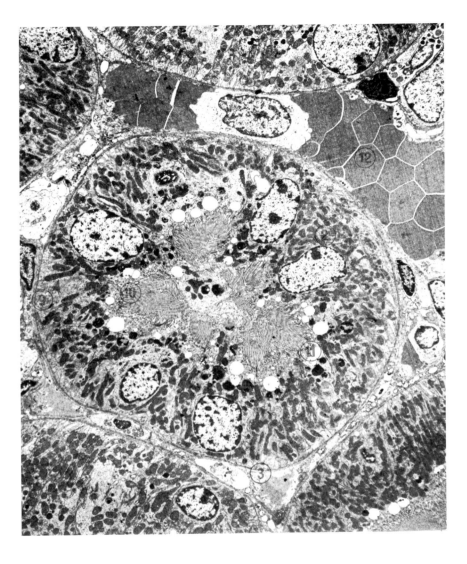

# Developmental Abnormalities

THE DEVELOPMENT of the human kidney is complex, involving a sequence of three primary structures—the pronephros, the mesonephros and the metanephros. Of these, the first two soon disappear leaving only duct remnants which are, however, important for the subsequent development of the metanephros which becomes the definitive adult kidney. The latter is derived from two primary tissues or anlages: (a) the nephrogenic blastema which gives rise to the nephrons including the renal corpuscles and (b) the ureteric bud which grows out from the mesonephric duct to form the ureter, pelvi-calyceal system and the collecting ducts within the kidney. During the sixth to eighth weeks of development the kidneys migrate from original pelvic to final lumbar positions and rotate through right angles to bring each renal hilus from a ventral to a medial relationship with the main kidney mass.

Normal kidney development requires not only the sequential formation and disappearance of the early primordial organs but the correct development and fusion of blastema with ureteric components of the metanephros. Failure to achieve this can produce a range of abnormalities including absence of a kidney (agenesis), abnormally fused or "horse-shoe" kidneys as well as a range of cystic changes; rarely, abnormally situated or ectopic kidneys may result. Variations in the number and anatomical course of the renal arteries, or their main segmental branches, quite commonly give rise to so-called accessory or aberrant vessels.

In this section, only some of the more common developmental anomalies are illustrated.

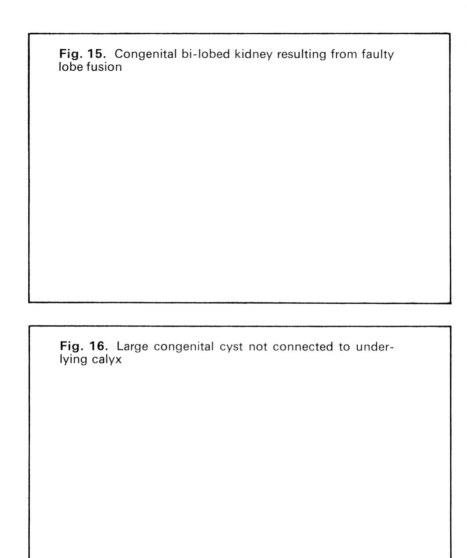

**Fig. 15.** Congenital bi-lobed kidney resulting from faulty lobe fusion

**Fig. 16.** Large congenital cyst not connected to underlying calyx

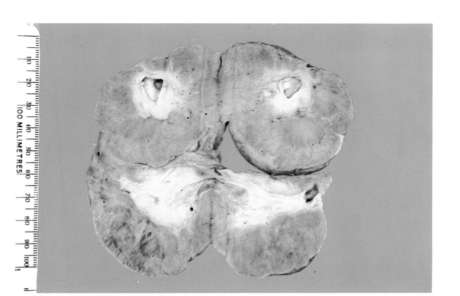

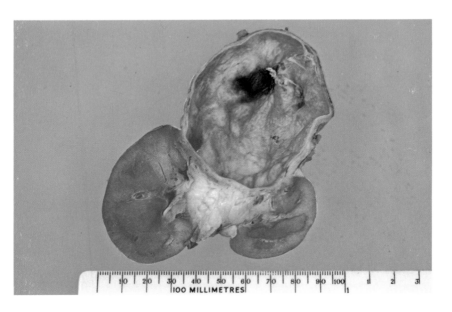

**Fig. 17.** "Adult-type" cystic disease in an infant kidney with "horse-shoe" deformity. Much of the kidney substance is replaced by small spherical cysts

**Fig. 18.** Polycystic disease in an adult: both the cut surface (*left*) and cortical surface show masses of thin-walled cysts

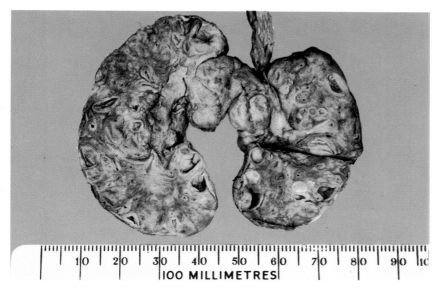

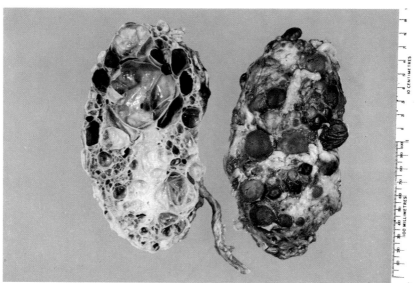

**Fig. 19.** Adult polycystic disease; cyst walls are formed of connective tissue lined with low cuboidal epithelium (H and E x 330)

**Fig. 20.** Adult polycystic disease; some cysts contain granular proteinous debris and red blood cells (MSB x 66)

**Fig. 21.** Adult polycystic disease: areas of calcification (*bottom centre*) occur in cyst walls and contents (H and E x 66)

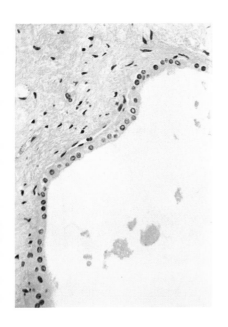

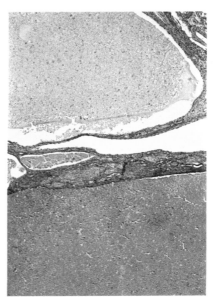

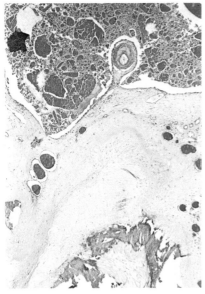

**Fig. 22.** Infantile polycystic disease; showing mass of fusiform cysts in kidney substance

**Fig. 23.** Infantile polycystic disease: showing elongated clefts or "cysts" with glomerular corpuscles within the walls (H and E x 66)

**Fig. 24.** Cystic dilatation of liver bile ducts from case illustrated in Figs. 22 and 23 (H and E x 154)

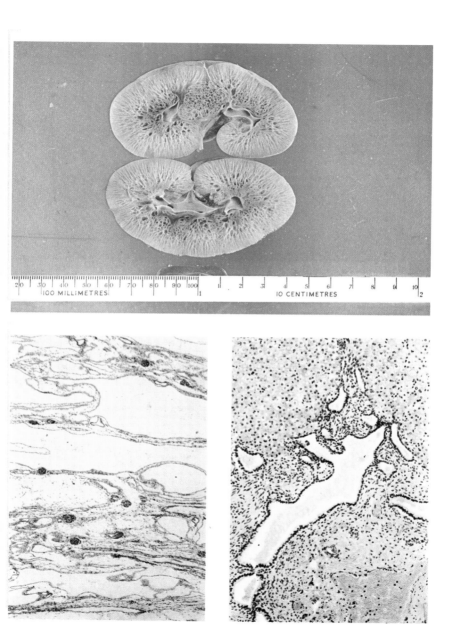

2|0   3|0   4|0   5|0   6|0   7|0   8|0   9|0   10|0   1   2   3   4   5   6   7   8   9   10   2
|100 MILLIMETRES|                                    10 CENTIMETRES

**Fig. 25.** Form of medullary sponge kidney: cyst formation in the medulla and renal papillae. Specimen obtained from a 42-year-old male patient who died from cancer of large intestine

**Fig. 26.** Medullary sponge kidney: the cysts represent dilated collecting ducts (H and E x 66)

**Fig. 27.** Medullary sponge kidney: cysts are lined with flat cuboidal epithelium (H and E x 330)

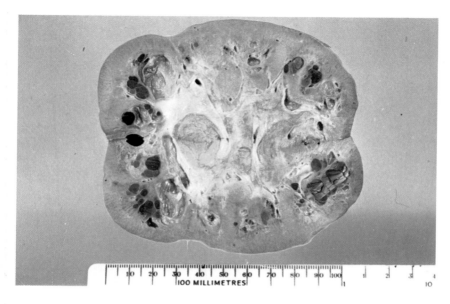

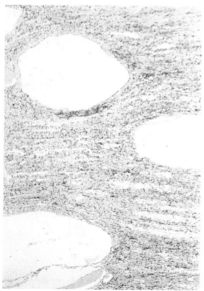
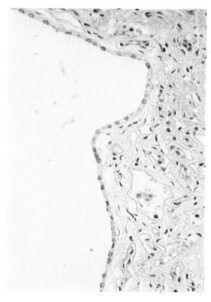

**Fig. 28.** Abnormal kidney development resulting in pelvis and ureter arising from lateral aspect of kidney (*left*) whilst main renal artery (*arrowed*) enters lower renal pole as a branch of the common iliac artery

**Fig. 29.** Ectopic adrenal tissue (*arrowed*) below renal capsule. The kidney has been injected with a blue dye to increase colour contrast

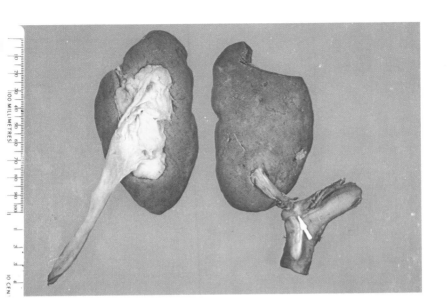

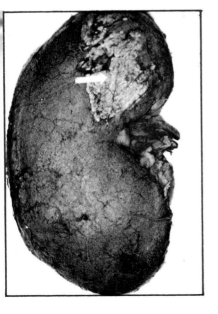

# Renal Infection

PATHOGENIC ORGANISMS may enter the kidney by the blood stream or by retrograde spread along the ureter or peri-ureteric lymphatics from a primary infection in the lower urinary tract. Blood-borne organisms, e.g., staphylococci, are usually confined to the kidney substance (parenchyma) where they may produce pyaemic abscesses. Organisms (mainly of coliform types) entering by the ureteric pathways may produce infection of the pelvi-calyceal system as a pyelitis, or, more commonly, extend outwards to involve the parenchyma as a pyelonephritis.

Pyelonephritis may be acute or chronic and affect either or both kidneys; acute attacks may be repeated, particularly when there is interference to urine drainage by stones, tumours, an enlarged prostate, or by the physiological loss of tone which often affects the ureters in pregnancy.

Acute pyelonephritis causes swelling of the kidneys; the mucosa of the pelvi-calyces is congested and yellow streaks radiating outwards from the pelvis indicate the pathways of spreading infection throughout the parenchyma where abscesses may be formed.

In chronic pyelonephritis the kidneys are usually smaller than normal—sometimes markedly so—and their shape is distorted by coarse fibrous scars which replace lost or damaged nephrons. Areas of normal kidney tissue lie between the scars, but in some cases the chronic inflammation may affect the organ diffusely. Foci of acute inflammation may be superimposed on the chronic changes. Surviving tubules may compensate by enlargement and are dilated with protein casts. Rarely the disease may assume a granulomatous form. Patients with chronic pyelonephritis tend to develop increased blood pressure which produces characteristic changes in the renal arteries. When both kidneys are severely involved, failure of renal function is common and progressive.

Tuberculous infection is always secondary to extra-renal tuberculosis, e.g., in lung. Widely scattered blood-borne bacilli produce many small focal (miliary) lesions, or lodge in the medullary apices where caseous necrosis leads to ulceration and cavitation.

Viral infections of specific renal importance are rare. Cyto-megalic inclusion disease, more common in young children and probably of viral origin, results in giant cell formation by the renal tubular epithelium. These giant cell forms have characteristic "inclusions" in either their nuclei or cytoplasm.

**Fig. 30.** Pyaemic abscesses appear as small yellow spots with dark margins throughout cortex and medulla. The abscesses resulted from a blood-borne staphylococcal infection

**Fig. 31.** Pyaemic abscesses appear as circumscribed cellular foci in the cortex (H and E x 66)

**Fig. 32.** Pus cells represented by polymorph leucocytes, and macrophages within pyaemic abscess (H and E x 330)

**Fig. 33.** Dark mass represents bacterial colonies within abscess (H and E x 550)

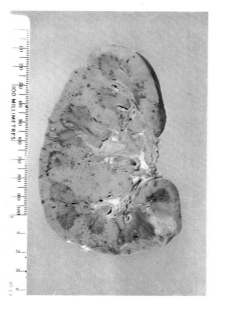

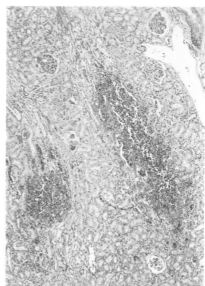

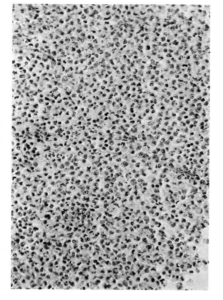

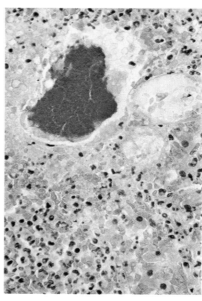

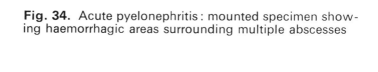
**Fig. 34.** Acute pyelonephritis: mounted specimen showing haemorrhagic areas surrounding multiple abscesses

**Fig. 35.** Acute pyelonephritis following surgical anastomosis of ureter to intestinal loop and total cystectomy for bladder cancer

**Fig. 36.** Acute pyelonephritis: radial (blue) streaks in medulla and cortex indicate pathways of infection (H and E x 1)

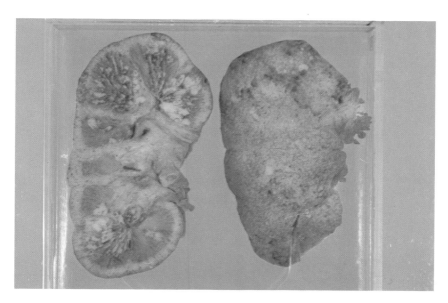

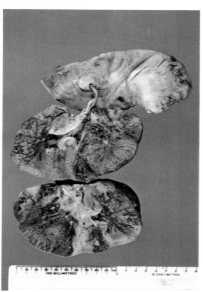

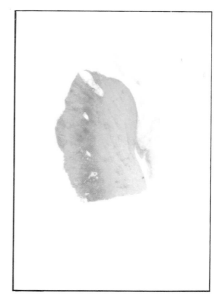

**Fig. 37.** Pus and red cells in collecting tubules in acute pyelonephritis (H and E x 66)

**Fig. 38.** Acute pyelonephritis showing areas of acute interstitial inflammation (H and E x 352)

**Fig. 39.** Abscess formation and surrounding interstitial inflammation in acute pyelonephritis (MSB x 66)

**Fig. 40.** Acute pyelonephritis showing pus and organisms in disrupted tubules (H and E x 550)

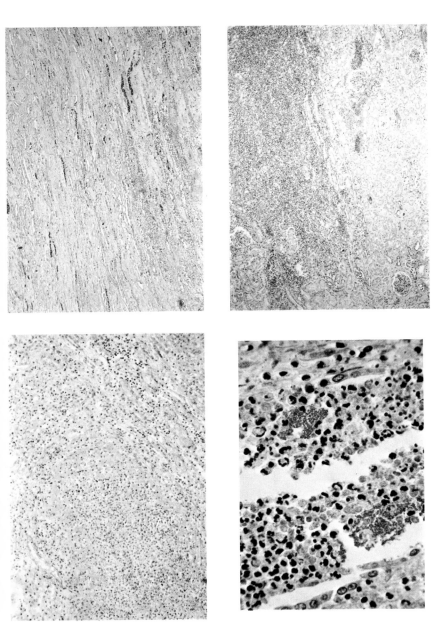

**Fig. 41.** Chronic pyelonephritis : normal kidney (*left*) contrasts with severely scarred, contracted kidney of chronic pyelonephritis (*right*)

**Fig. 42.** Kidney pelvis is thickened by fibrous tissue and chronic inflammation; the overlying mucosa has lost part of its epithelial lining (H and E x 110)

**Fig. 43.** Chronic pyelonephritis showing dense interstitial inflammation, sclerosis of glomeruli and loss of tubules (MSB x 143)

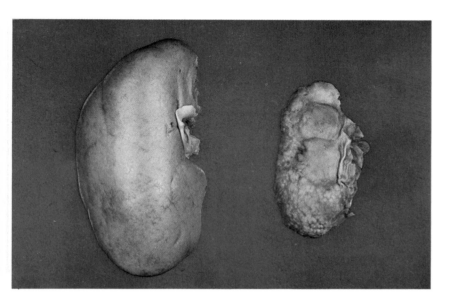

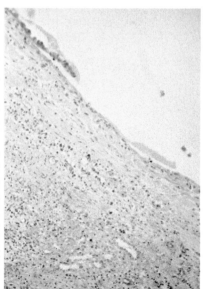

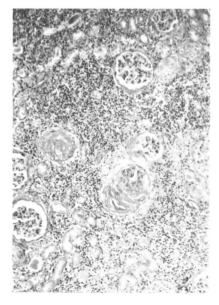

**Fig. 44.** Hyaline thickening of capsular membranes and dense inflammatory infiltrate around glomeruli in chronic pyelonephritis (H and E x 330)

**Fig. 45.** Peri-capsular fibrosis and glomerular atrophy in chronic pyelonephritis (H and E x 330)

**Fig. 46.** Severe parenchymal atrophy in chronic pyelonephritis showing hyalinised glomeruli, tubular loss and interstitial fibrosis. Occasional tubules are dilated with proteinous casts (H and E x 154)

**Fig. 47.** "Thyroid-like" areas in chronic pyelonephritis comprising tubules dilated with protein casts (red) (MSB x 154)

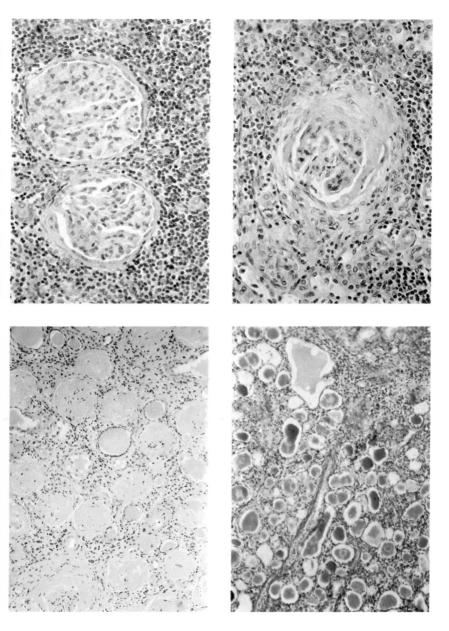

**Fig. 48.** Woven bone formation in renal papilla in a case of chronic pyelonephritis, partially polarised (H and E x 154)

**Fig. 49.** Adenomatous tubular hyperplasia in chronic pyelonephritis (H and E x 330)

**Fig. 50.** Neutral fat in hyalinised glomerulus and periglomerular fibrous tissue (Oil red O—haematoxylin x 330)

**Fig. 51.** Xanthogranulomatous form of chronic pyelonephritis. There is extensive necrosis of kidney tissue and reactive fibrosis. Appearances suggest tuberculous caseation, but it is not of tuberculous origin

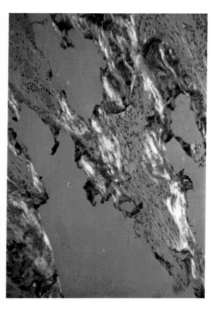
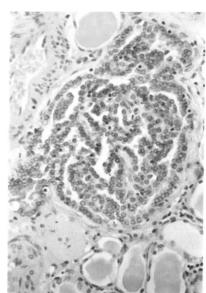
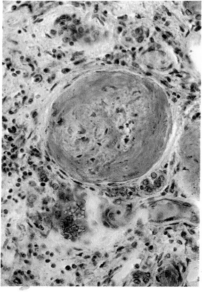
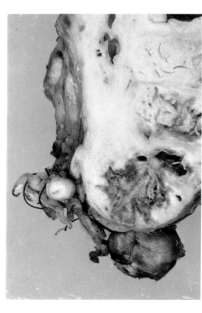

**Fig. 52.** Another example of xanthogranulomatous chronic pyelonephritis associated with hydronephrosis and cortical cysts

**Fig. 53.** Giant cell macrophages are a feature of this condition. Tissue taken from specimen shown in Fig. 51 (H and E x 330)

**Fig. 54.** Chronic pyelonephritis associated with kidney calculus. Most of the kidney tissue has been destroyed by infection and replaced by fat. There was also a pyonephrosis and perinephric abscess. A portion of supra-renal tissue remains above the upper pole

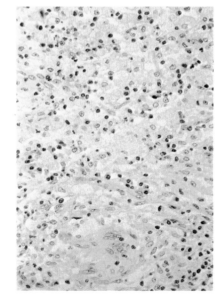

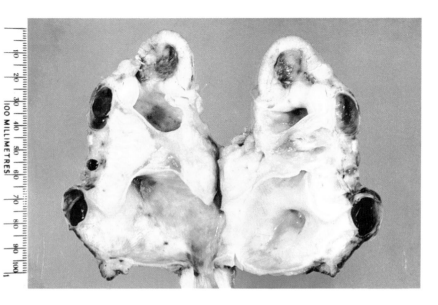

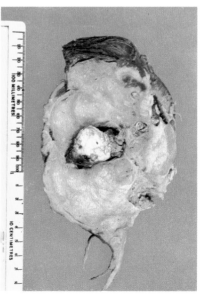

**Fig. 55.** Ulceration and inflammation of renal pelvis with pus in pelvic cavity (*left*). Tissue taken from specimen shown in Fig. 54 (MSB x 66)

**Fig. 56.** Chronic pyelonephritis showing muscular hypertrophy of arcuate and interlobular arteries indicative of hypertension (PAS x 66)

**Fig. 57.** Tuberculous pyelonephritis: several tuberculous follicles with giant cell systems occur throughout the cortex which is diffusely but densely infiltrated with chronic inflammatory cells. Glomeruli are identifiable but there is severe tubular loss (H and E x 66)

**Fig. 58.** Same case as illustrated in Fig. 57 showing larger area of tuberculous caseous necrosis (*bottom left*) (H and E x 66)

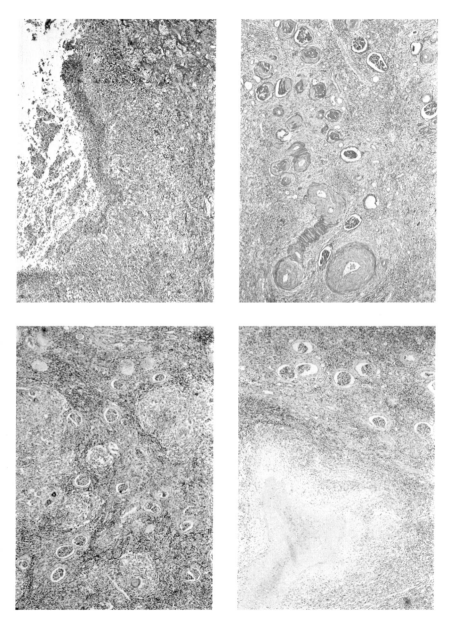

**Fig. 59.** Tuberculous pyelonephritis: part of a tuberculous follicle showing mainly peripheral lymphocytes (*upper half*) and epitheloid cells with giant cell formation (*lower right and centre*) (H and E x 154)

**Fig. 60.** Advanced renal tuberculosis: the kidney tissue has been extensively replaced by caseous necrotic debris which also distends the proximal ureter

**Fig. 61.** Woven bone formation in long standing tuberculous infection.
Around the bone convexity there is caseous debris; in its concavity there is attempt to form bone marrow (partially polarised) (H and E x 165)

**Fig. 62.** Long standing renal tuberculosis; a thin rim of remaining cortex (*above*) is separated from a caseous area (*below*) by a band of fibrous tissue (H and E x 66)

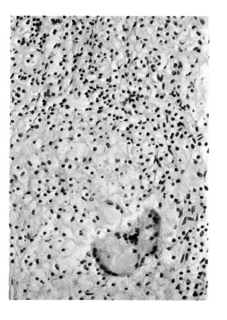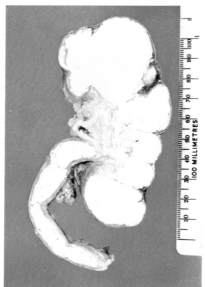
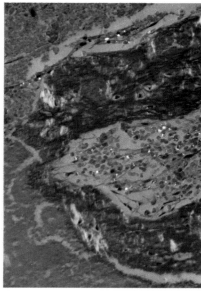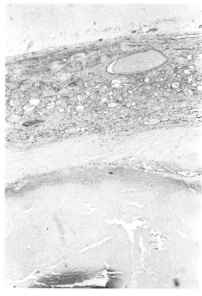

**Fig. 63.** Tuberculous pyelitis: the mucosa of the kidney pelvis has been replaced by a zone of inflammatory tissue (*left*). The underlying stroma shows tuberculous follicle formation (*right*) (H and E x 66)

**Fig. 64.** Cytomegalic inclusion disease in an infant. The renal tubule is lined by giant cells with characteristic "inclusions" (H and E x 330)

**Fig. 65.** Higher magnification of basophilic intranuclear and intracytoplasmic inclusions in tubular epithelium (H and E x 550)

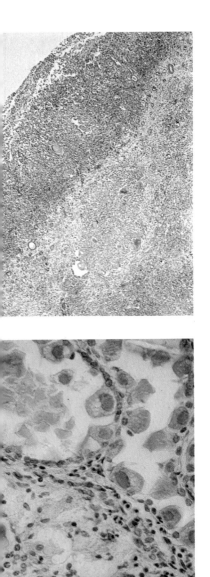
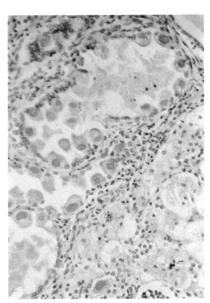

# Vascular Disturbances

### Renal infarction

Renal infarction, a coagulative ischaemic necrosis of the kidney, most often results from blockage of the arterial blood supply. This may be due to thrombosis—alone or in combination with atheroma or necrotising arteritis—to embolism, arterial injury or to severe arterial spasm. Thrombosis of the renal vein is a rare cause, seen mostly in infants as a complication of dehydration. Renal infarcts vary in size and number relative to causal mechanisms and to the size and number of blocked vessels.

The sequence of tissue changes within an infarct cannot be followed in man, as in experimental animals, but evidence from both sources supports a common interpretation. A recent infarct forms a dark red, wedge-shaped area mainly within the cortex but its apex may penetrate the medulla. In its centre vessels and glomeruli are congested but cell nuclei remain for several days. Tissue damage is at first most severe towards the periphery of the infarct whose outer limits are marked by narrow haemorrhagic margins. After a few days, the centre becomes pale with breakdown of the red blood cells. In small infarcts polymorph leucocyte infiltration may be diffuse but never dense; in large infarcts, though transient, it is often concentrated around the necrotic central mass. Later, in the marginal congested zone, some damaged tubules are re-epithelialised, others die and, together with reactive connective tissue, form the final boundary between infarct and healthy kidney tissue. Infarcts shrink slowly with collapse and fusion of their central dead tissue which may partially calcify but retain their outlines for many months.

*Emboli*, which cause infarcts, consist of particles of solid material (e.g., broken off fragments of thrombi). Other and less common forms which may involve the kidney—often at glomerular level—include fat droplets following bone fractures or injury to subcutaneous fatty tissue, lipids and cholesterol from ulcerated atheromatous plaques, and occasionally groups of malignant cells as a form of tumour spread.

The most dramatic form of renal infarction—*renal cortical necrosis*—occurs mainly as a rare complication of pregnancy in association with placental apoplexy. Of vaso-spastic origin, and sometimes complicated by thrombosis within the spastic arteries, the lesion varies in severity from small focal infarcts to extensive confluent necrosis of the cortices of both kidneys. In severe fatal forms, the kidneys are swollen—the pale, necrotic cortices contrasting with the haemorrhagic medullae. Limited focal forms are not fatal, the infarcts undergoing repair.

## Arteriosclerosis and hypertension

Changes of a biochemical and structural nature, referred to as arteriosclerosis, affect arteries with increasing age independent of patients' blood pressure levels. In the kidneys these changes are best seen in the muscular arteries down to arcuate level and appear as thickening of their intimal lining by fibro-elastic tissue and some fibrosis of their medial coats. This produces gradual shrinkage of kidney parenchyma with some hyalinisation of arterioles and glomeruli, atrophy of tubules (mainly proximal ones), increase of interstitital connective tissue and variable lymphocytic infiltration. Renal function is not significantly impaired.

## Hypertension

Most cases of high blood pressure are of the essential type. A few are secondary to other conditions of which renal ischaemia is the most common. The degree of hypertension may be moderate and remain so for many years as a *benign* form, or severe, in a *malignant* form and of short duration. Both affect the kidneys in different ways.

*Benign hypertension* often accentuates the changes of arteriosclerosis, with reduction in cortical width and fine granularity of subcapsular surfaces. Eosinophilic hyaline material is prominent in the walls of arterioles (mainly afferent ones), in glomerular capillaries and sometimes within their capsules which are thickened by fibrous tissue. The proportion of damaged glomeruli and atrophied nephrons varies in different cases; groups of surviving tubules may enlarge and dilate to compensate functionally for those lost, but the loss of kidney tissue is never severe enough to produce renal failure.

*Malignant hypertension* usually follows a benign phase; thus kidney size varies. In rare cases, when malignant hypertension arises *de novo*, the kidneys are swollen and haemorrhagic; their cortical surfaces are smooth and mottled. About a third of their glomeruli and supplying arterioles are destroyed by fibrinoid necrosis and smaller muscular arteries (mainly interlobular) are concentrically narrowed by loose mucoid connective tissue.

Hypertension secondary to *renal ischaemia* may result from stenosis of a main renal artery by atheroma, thrombosis within aneurysms of the main renal arteries or, rarely, from fibro-muscular hypertrophy of the arterial muscular coats. These types of stenosis are usually unilateral and theoretically amenable to surgical correction, but long term results of surgical repair tend to be disappointing. Renal ischaemia probably also underlies the hypertension which complicates other renal diseases, e.g., glomerulonephritis, pyelonephritis and hydronephrosis.

**Fig. 66.** Numerous recent cortical infarcts (*arrowed*) produced by emboli from cardiac mural thrombus

**Fig. 67.** Slightly older cortical infarct appearing as wedge-shaped pale area with narrow surrounding haemorrhagic zone

**Fig. 68.** Infarcts retain their cell nuclei for several days (H and E x 143)

**Fig. 69.** Narrow cellular zone separates infarct (*left*) from adjacent viable but congested kidney tissue (*right*) (Trichrome x 66)

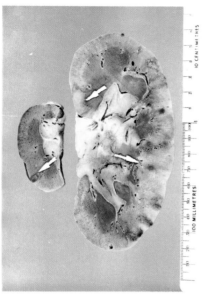

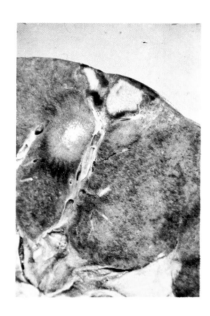

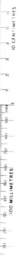

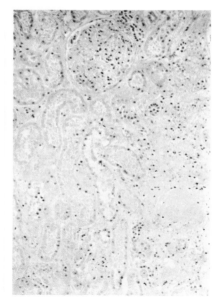

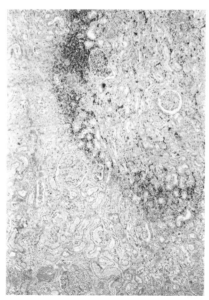

**Fig. 70.** Regeneration of tubular epithelium in peripheral reactive zone around renal infarct. A tubular cell in mitosis appears in lower right corner (H and E x 330)

**Fig. 71.** With ageing, infarct gradually loses its colour and undergoes contraction (*see centre left cortex*)

**Fig. 72.** Old infarcts producing areas of contraction and scarring of cortex

**Fig. 73.** Old healed infarct. The infarct (*right*) is covered by a thickened kidney capsule (*left*) (H and E x 66)

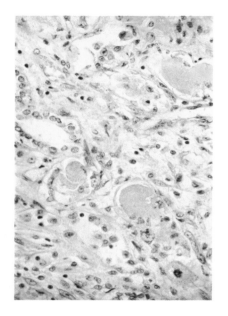

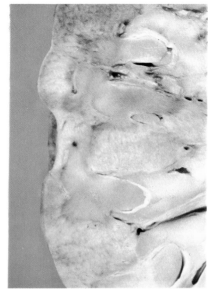

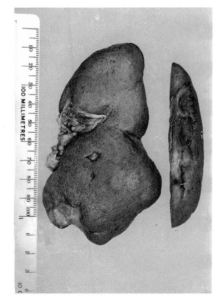

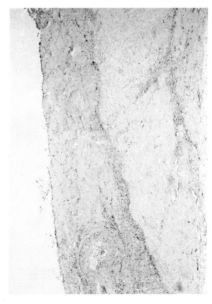

**Fig. 74.** Severe loss of kidney substance as a result of ischaemia produced by thrombosis of renal artery (see Fig. x 75)

**Fig. 75.** Renal artery from specimen illustrated in Fig. 74, showing lumen occluded by organised thrombus (PAS x 66)

**Fig. 76.** Ischaemic atrophy of cortical parenchyma in specimen illustrated in Figs. 74 and 75 (PAS x 66)

**Fig. 77.** Fibrin micro-emboli lodged in glomerular capillaries following graft repair of an abdominal aortic aneurysm. The capillaries involved lie to the left and below centre towards the vascular pole (H and E x 330)

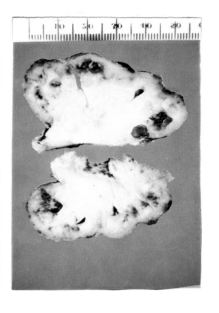

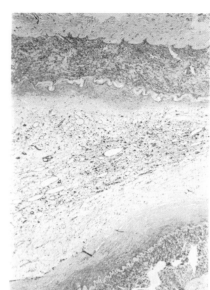

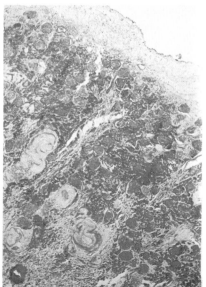

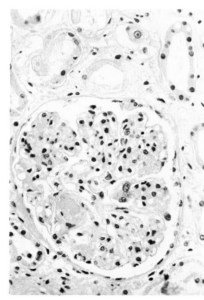

**Fig. 78.** Fat emboli in glomerular capillaries following multiple bone fractures. The fat is represented by "empty" spaces in the capillary lumina, following processing of tissue in fat solvents (H and E x 330)

**Fig. 79.** Larger embolus lodged in arcuate artery at the apex of infarct. The embolus consists of fibrin (red) and blood cells (Trichrome x 154)

**Fig. 80.** Renal vein thrombosis. The vein issuing from the renal hilum is totally occluded

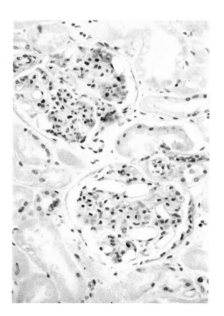

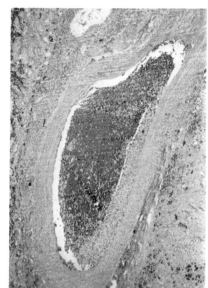

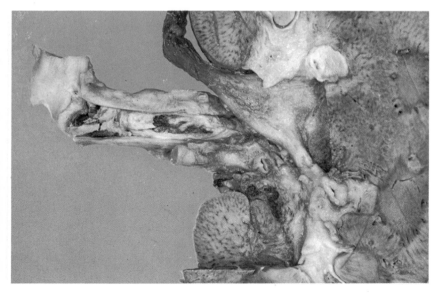

**Fig. 81.** Transverse section of renal vein shown in Fig. 80. The vessel lumen is occupied by laminated thrombus (MSB x 66)

**Fig. 82.** Renal vein thrombosis. Glomerular and intertubular capillaries are acutely congested with blood, but there is no infarction (MSB x 330)

**Fig. 83.** Peri-renal haematoma resulting from a road traffic accident. The red/brown zone (*left*) represents unorganised blood clot; the central area is occupied by organising tissue which contains abundant brown iron pigment (H and E x 96)

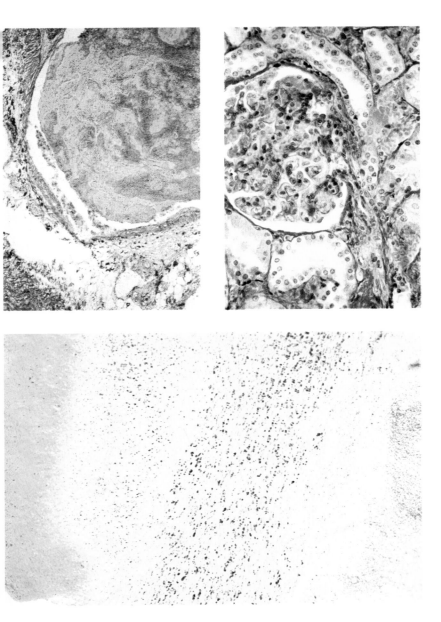

**Fig. 84.** Renal cortical necrosis. There is extensive confluent necrosis of cortex which appears pale, surrounding the congested medulla

**Fig. 85.** Confluent bilateral cortical necrosis complicating septic endometritis

**Fig. 86.** Edge of cortical necrotic zone showing necrosis of tubules and glomeruli (*bottom*). Recent thrombus occupies the lumen of arcuate and interlobular arteries (MSB x 66)

**Fig. 87.** Focal form of cortical necrosis with damage confined to small areas in which there is thrombosis of glomerular capillaries and limited tubular loss (H and E x 154)

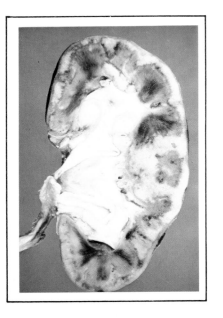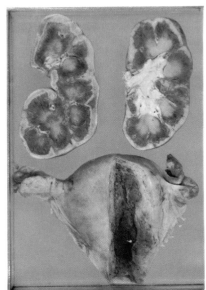

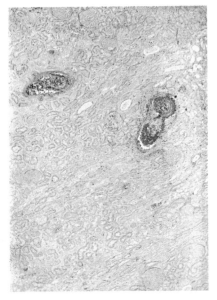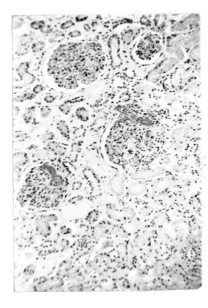

**Fig. 88.** Arteriosclerosis in an elderly normotensive subject. There is thickening of walls of small muscular arteries with laminar reduplication of elastic tissue (EVG x 264)

**Fig. 89.** Atherosclerosis of renal artery showing eccentric intimal plaque containing lipid (Oil red O-Haematoxylin x 11)

**Fig. 90.** Atherosclerosis—a form of arteriosclerosis in which lipids and cholesterol are laid down in arterial lining —producing significant narrowing of the renal artery (*arrowed*). The cortex is narrowed as a result of renal ischaemia

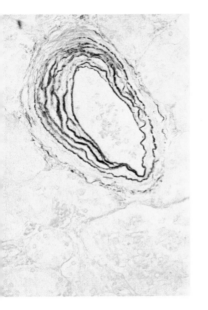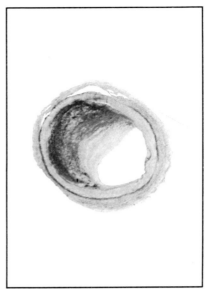

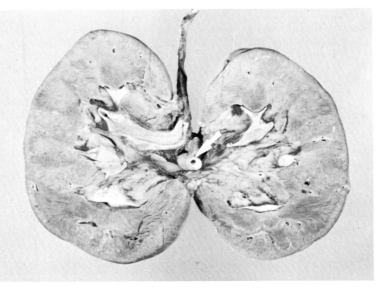

**Fig. 91.** Benign hypertension. The kidney shows moderate narrowing of its cortex, prominence of arteries and a finely granular cortical surface on removing the kidney capsule

**Fig. 92.** Benign hypertension showing a coarser cortical scarring and several cortical cysts. There is also severe atheroma of the aorta and its principal branches

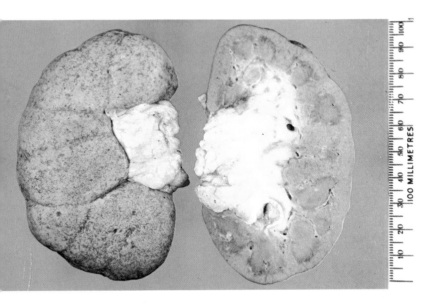

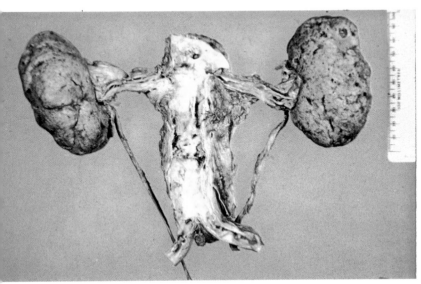

**Fig. 93.** In benign hypertension there is hyalinisation of arteriole walls—seen here in red; red blood cells in adjacent capillaries appear yellow (MSB x 308)

**Fig. 94.** Patchy tubular atrophy and glomerular sclerosis are common features of benign hypertension (MSB x 66)

**Fig. 95.** Some tubules are dilated with pink colloid (proteinous) casts. Benign hypertension (H and E x 330)

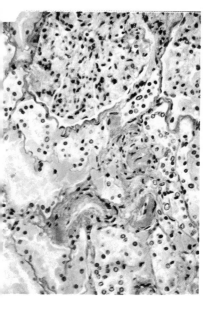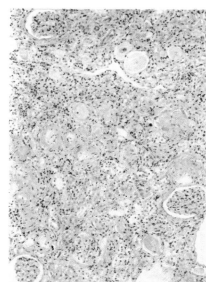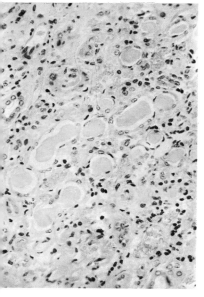

**Fig. 96.** Malignant hypertension. The kidney is swollen and shows haemorrhagic mottling of its surfaces. There is also haemorrhage into pelvi-calyces

**Fig. 97.** Fibrinoid necrosis of glomerular capillaries in malignant hypertension produces blurring of capillary outlines and allows haemorrhages into the urinary space (H and E x 374)

**Fig. 98.** Malignant hypertension: showing fibrinoid necrosis of arterioles and glomerular capillaries (red), and intra-tubular haemorrhages (yellow) above glomerulus (MSB x 132)

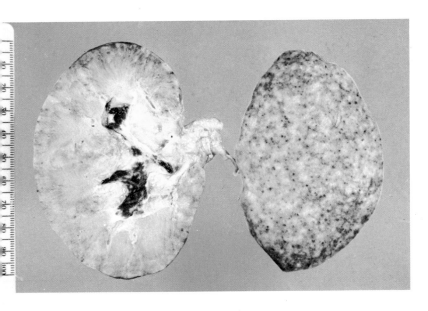

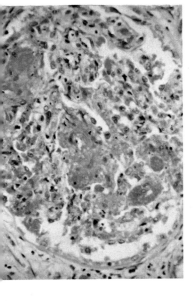

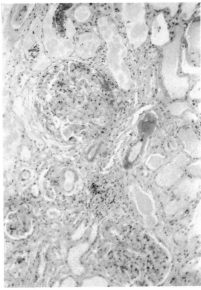

**Fig. 99.** Malignant hypertension showing patchy loss of tubules (lower half) and compensatory dilatation of others (upper half) (MSB x 55)

**Fig. 100.** Lower nephron tubules often contain haemorrhagic or colloid casts in malignant hypertension (H and E x 55)

**Fig. 101.** Severe hypertension treated with hypotensive drugs. There is serious parenchymal damage and prominent intimal thickening of small muscular arteries seen in cross-section (PAS x 55)

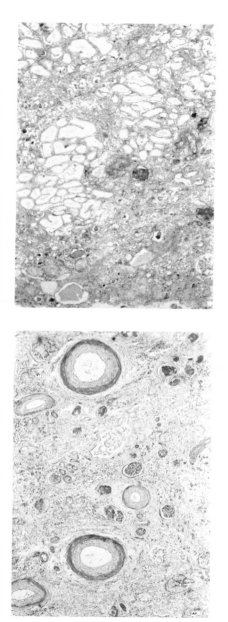
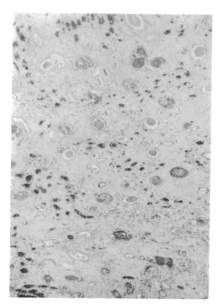

# Glomerular Disease and the Nephrotic Syndrome

THE GLOMERULUS reacts to harmful stimuli in a limited number of ways. Damage may affect the epithelial cells, capillary basement membranes, the mesangium, endothelium or combinations of these structures. Should this occur in the absence of other systematised disease, it is referred to as glomerulonephritis—a disease which can assume a variety of forms. In some patients it causes heavy proteinuria, hypoalbuminaemia, fluid retention and raised levels of serum cholesterol—a clinical condition referred to as *the nephrotic syndrome*. In others it produces a short illness with proteinuria, mild haematuria, oedema and hypertension from which the majority recover completely. In both categories, however, a proportion of patients fail to recover, becoming increasingly ill with raised levels of blood urea, dehydration, acidosis, anaemia and variable hypertension—indicating chronic renal failure—a fatal condition unless relieved by dialysis or renal transplantation.

Knowledge of glomerulonephritis (more accurately termed glomerular disease) has been increased by the study of renal biopsies which allows correlation of the tissue changes with the clinical signs or syndromes they produce. The causes of the glomerular damage vary; some are unknown, others take the form of immune (antigen-antibody) complexes or anti-basement membrane antibodies laid down within glomerular capillary basement membranes. It is now clear that this category of renal disease is primarily of glomerular and not of tubular origin. In the classification which follows, therefore, descriptions of tissue changes are restricted to the glomerulus, the associated tubular or interstitial ones being regarded as secondary although they may be extensive and important.

# CLASSIFICATION OF GLOMERULONEPHRITIS

**Note:** LM—Light microscopical; EM—Electron microscopical; Im—Immunological reaction; Ig—Immune globulin; b.m.—basement membrane.

| TYPE | MAIN CLINICAL FEATURES | MAIN GLOMERULAR CHANGES |
|---|---|---|
| **1.** *Minimal change:* | affects mainly children; microscopic haematuria.; nephrotic syndrome—responds to steroids; usually good prognosis; rarely progresses to renal failure. | LM: no change apart from mild hypercellularity.<br>EM: basement membranes normal; fusion of epithelial cell foot processes.<br>Im: small deposits of IgE have been reported in b.m. |
| **2.** *Idiopathic membranous:* | affects mainly adults; insidious onset of proteinuria leading to nephrotic syndrome; poor prognosis—slow progression to renal failure. | LM: B.m. diffusely thickened—epi-membranous "spikes" in silver stained sections.<br>EM: amorphous deposits and lucent areas in the b.m.<br>Im: immune complexes and sometimes complement in b.m. |

**3.** *Diffuse proliferative:*  affects mainly children or young adults following infection with Group A haemolytic streptococci or other organisms.

(a) Acute type

albuminuria; haematuria; oedema; mild hypertension; majority recover completely; a minority progress to (b) or (c).

LM: hypercellularity; increase in intrinsic cells, polymorph leucocytes and macrophages.
EM: electron dense "humps" in outer b.m. layers.
Im: immune complexes and complement in b.m.

(b) Rapidly progressive type

haematuria; albuminuria; granular/cellular urine casts; renal failure; hypertension; sometimes nephrotic syndrome; poor prognosis.

LM: hypercellularity and lobulation of tufts with capsular adhesions and capsular crescents; occasional necrosis in fatal cases.
EM: hypercellularity; some increase of b.m. thickness and b.m. material within mesangium.

(c) Slowly progressive type

affects mainly middle age group; renal failure; hypertension; poor prognosis; renal osteodystrophy.

LM: hyalinisation of vascular tufts; concentric fibrosis within capsules.
EM: confirms LM appearances.
Im: Ig, complement and fibrin in variable amount and distribution.

**4.** *Membrano-proliferative*

and


Cause unknown; haematuria, hypocomplement-aemia, nephrotic syndrome—response to steroids, immuno-suppression and anti-coagulants under investigation.

LM/EM: patchy b.m. thickening; sub-endothelial de-position of mesangial matrix along b.m.; in-crease in mesangial cells; dense deposits in b.m.
Im: Ig in b.m. and mesangium.

*Chronic lobular variant*

LM/EM: lobulation of tufts resulting from excess matrix production.

**5.** *Focal*
(a) *proliferative*

haematuria, variable albuminuria: prognosis depends on cause.

LM/EM: cellular proliferation in proportion of tufts or tuft segments.
Im: Ig, complement and fibrin deposition.

(b) *sclerosing*

absence of systemic disease; haematuria, nephrotic syndrome.

LM/EM: segmental or total sclerosis of tufts without cell-ular proliferation beginning in juxta-medullary glomeruli.

Fig. 102. "Minimal change" type glomerulonephritis. No structural change is detectable in this glomerular corpuscle by light microscopy although the patient concerned suffered from a nephrotic syndrome (MSB x 224)

Fig. 103. "Minimal change" type glomerulonephritis. There is slight prominence of mesangial cells but no other detectable abnormality. Capillary basement membranes are of normal thickness (PAS x 512)

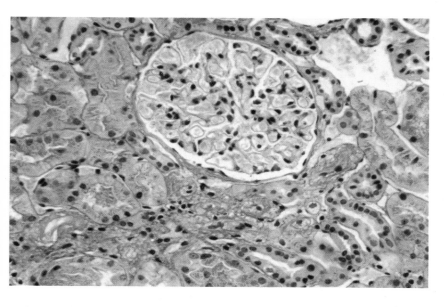
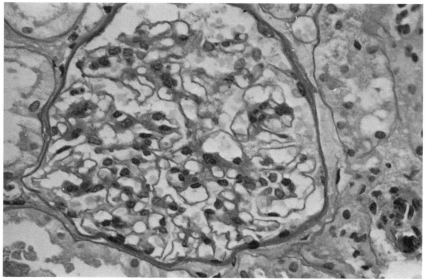

**Fig. 104.** Electron micrograph of "minimal change" type glomerulonephritis. The major abnormality is the fusion and collapse of epithelial foot processes (*arrowed*) along outer aspect of capillary basement membrane which is of normal thickness. The endothelial lining appears normal.

2—epithelial cell cytoplasm
3—basement membrane
4—red blood cell in capillary lumen
6—endothelial lining
(x 10,750 nm)

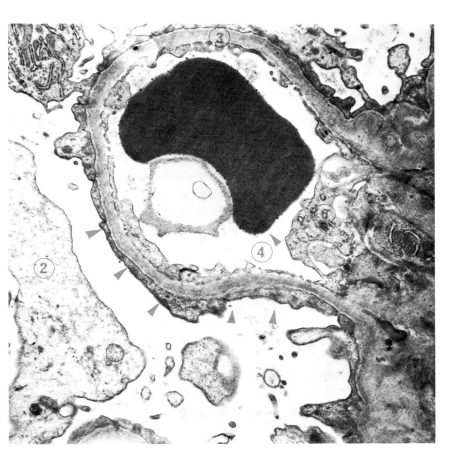

**Fig. 105.** Idiopathic membranous glomerulonephritis. The kidney is enlarged and on section shows a characteristic pallor of its cortex in contrast with the darker medulla

**Fig. 106.** Idiopathic membranous glomerulonephritis. The main abnormality is the uniform thickening of capillary basement membranes. Compare with Fig. 102 (MSB x 224)

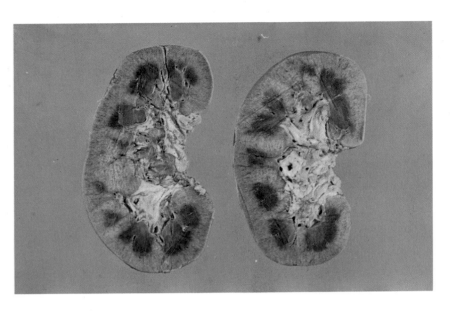

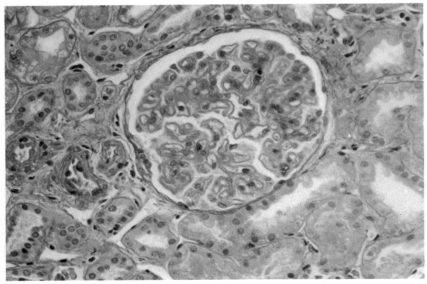

**Fig. 107.** For light microscopic diagnosis, basement membrane thickening can more easily be demonstrated in thin sections stained with silver (MeS x 330)

**Fig. 108.** Idiopathic membranous glomerulonephritis. Thicker section of glomerular capillary loops showing thickened basement membranes with characteristic "spike" projections along their epi-membranous borders (MeS x 1496)

**Fig. 109.** Idiopathic membranous glomerulonephritis. Cryostat section treated with fluorescent-labelled antiserum to IgG. Glomerular immune complexes emit a bright fluorescence with u/V excitation (x 480)

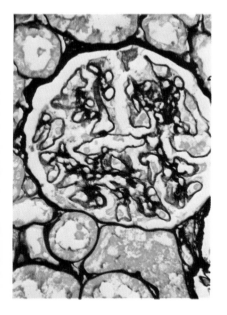
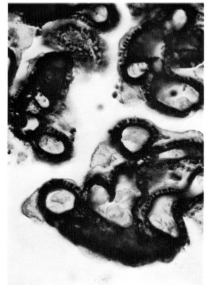
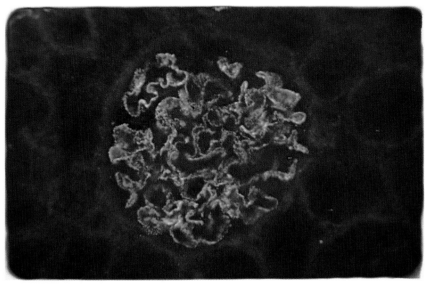

**Fig. 110.** Idiopathic membranous glomerulone-phritis. Electron micrograph of glomerular capillary loop showing markedly thickened basement membrane; electron-dense deposits (*arrowed*) in its outer zone represent deposits of antigen-antibody complexes. Intervening "clear" areas in the membrane correspond to the metalophil "spikes" seen in Fig. 108. The epithelial cell foot processes along outer border are fused

    3—basement membrane
    5—epithelial cell foot processes
    6—endothelial lining cell
    13—mesangium
    (x 10,750 nm)

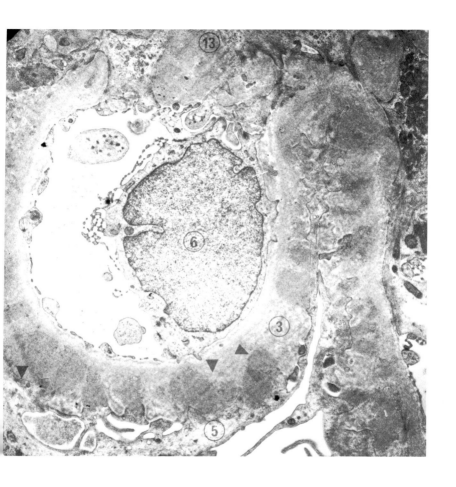

**Fig. 111.** Diffuse proliferative glomerulonephritis (acute phase). Glomeruli show increased cellularity and fill much of Bowman's space (H and E x 66)

**Fig. 112.** Increased cellularity of glomerulus in acute proliferative glomerulonephritis. There are occasional polymorph leucocytes in capillary lumina (PAS x 330)

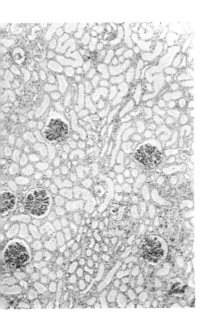 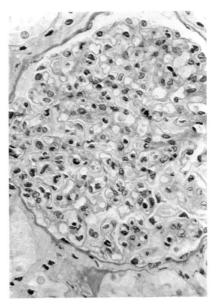

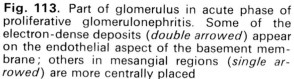

**Fig. 113.** Part of glomerulus in acute phase of proliferative glomerulonephritis. Some of the electron-dense deposits (*double arrowed*) appear on the endothelial aspect of the basement membrane; others in mesangial regions (*single arrowed*) are more centrally placed

    1—capillary lumen
    2—epithelial cell
    6—endothelial cell
    8—mesangial cell
    (x 7250 nm)

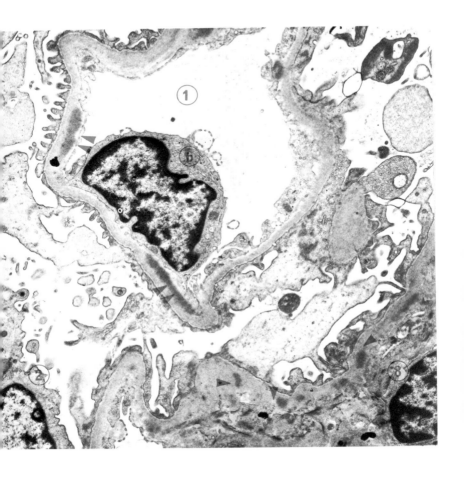

**Fig. 114.** Acute proliferative glomerulonephritis: cryostat section showing bright reaction in glomerulus to fluorescent-labelled anti-complement serum (x 330)

**Fig. 115.** Rapidly progressive diffuse glomerulonephritis. Glomerular outlines are obscured by adhesions to capsule and proliferation of capsular epithelium (MSB x 330)

**Fig. 116.** Glomerulus from case illustrated in Fig. 115, showing prominent capsular crescent (H and E x 330)

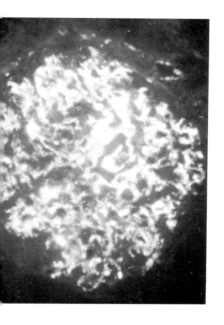

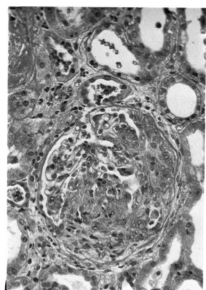

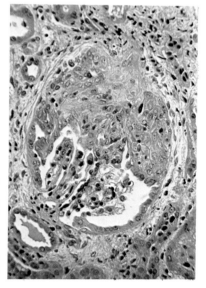

**Fig. 117.** Slowly progressive phase of diffuse glomerulo-nephritis. There is reduction of parenchyma, particulary of the cortex with increase in peri-pelvic fat content. The subcapsular surface is granular with cyst formation at one pole

**Fig. 118.** Section from kidney shown in Fig. 117. There is hyalinisation of glomeruli (some of which show capsular adhesions) and severe atrophy of tubules. The interstitium shows diffuse lymphocytic infiltration (H and E x 132)

**Fig. 119.** Slowly progressive proliferative glomerulo-nephritis(end-stage),showing advanced glomerular sclerosis and tubular damage (MSB x 66)

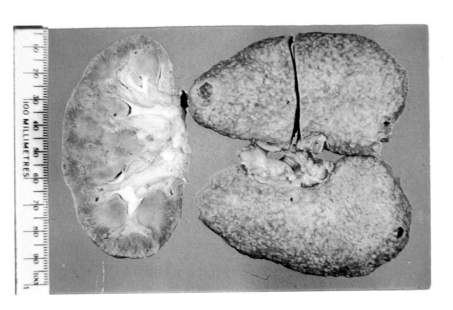

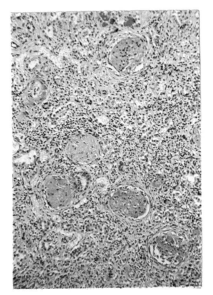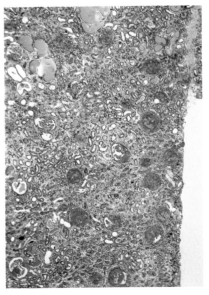

**Fig. 120.** Chronic lobular glomerulonephritis. There is a pronounced lobulation of glomerular tufts with excess of hyaline mesangial matrix. The patient presented with haematuria and nephrotic syndrome (PAS x 330)

**Fig. 121.** In lobular glomerulonephritis there is variable cellularity of the thickened mesangium. Cells tend to be distributed around the lobule periphere (MSB x 594)

**Fig. 122.** Focal proliferative glomerulonephritis. Three of the glomeruli show proliferative foci. Renal biopsy from a 29-year-old woman with clinical S.L.E. on steroid therapy (MSB x 132)

**Fig. 123.** Focal proliferative glomerulonephritis showing cellular proliferation and hyalinisation in lower glomerular lobules (PAS x 330)

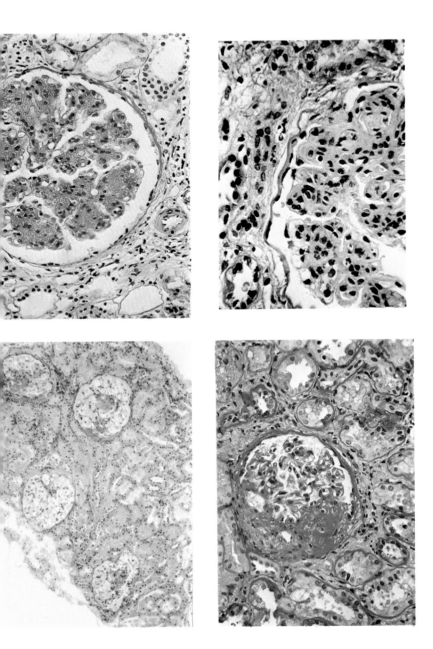

**Fig. 124.** Bright fluorescence obtained in glomerulus in focal glomerulonephritis with labelled anti-IgM globulin (x 330)

**Fig. 125.** Nephrotic syndrome associated with thrombosis of renal vein. The bisected kidney has a characteristic pale parenchyma; renal vein is occluded by thrombus

**Fig. 126.** Histology of specimen (Fig. 125) disclosed thickening of capillary basement membranes in all glomeruli, some of which also show capsular thickening with foam cell formation in epithelium (PAS x 330)

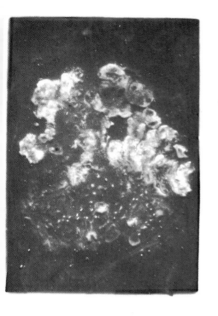 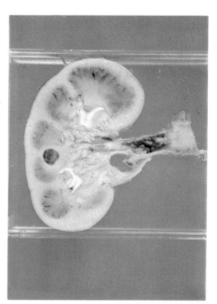

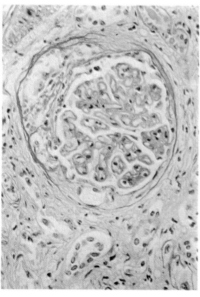

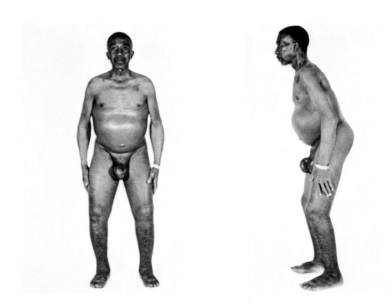

**Fig. 127.** Front and side views of an oedematous nephrotic patient. Fluid retention is particularly prominent in lower limbs, scrotum and abdomen, with protrusion of umbilicus

# Interstitial Nephritis

THIS DISEASE implies inflammatory involvement of the support-ing intertubular connective tissues in the absence of primary glomerular damage. The inflammation is not of bacterial origin nor primarily due to ischaemia although both factors may later complicate the disease.

In the acute form, interstitial nephritis may arise as an allergy to drugs, e.g., phenindione or sulphonamides, producing albumin-uria, oliguria or acute renal failure which may be fatal. In Britain, the chronic form may complicate high dosage with analgesics, particularly phenacetin. This produces interstitial inflammation, fibrosis and, in severe cases, a necrosis of the renal papillae. Clinical improvement usually follows withdrawal of the drug.

**Fig. 128.** Interstitial nephritis. Kidney is pale and swollen. There is a fine streaking of medulla and cortex denoting diffuse inflammation, and congestion of the pelvic mucosa. Patient was hypersensitive to phenindione

**Fig. 129.** Histology from kidney in Fig. 128 showing diffuse interstitial inflammation (H and E x 44)

**Fig. 130.** Interstitial nephritis. Glomeruli appear normal; inflammation is confined to inter-tubular tissue (H and E x 88)

**Fig. 131.** Higher magnification of part of Fig. 129 showing lymphocytes and occasional plasma cells in interstitial infiltrate. There is considerable tubular damage (H and E x 220)

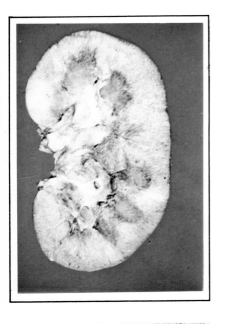

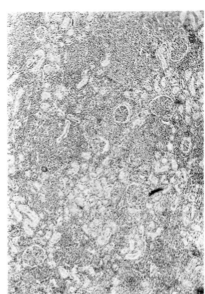

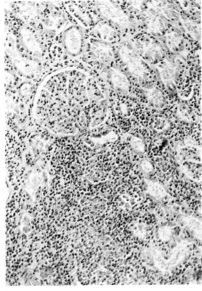

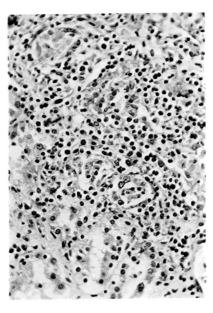

# The Nephropathies of Systemic Diseases

MANY DISEASES of extra-renal origin have important effects on renal structure and function. From this large group the following are considered in this section:

Group I: Diabetes mellitus and gout.

Group II: Systemic lupus erythematosus (S.L.E.), poly-arteritis nodosa, systemic sclerosis and Good-pasture's syndrome.

Group III: Amyloidosis, myelomatosis and Waldenström's macroglobulinaemia, sickle cell disease and leukaemia.

## GROUP I

### Diabetes Mellitus

*Pathological changes:* Glomeruli, arterioles and tubules are directly involved. Indirect effects include an increased incidence of pyelonephritis, necrotising papillitis and atherosclerosis of muscular (e.g., arcuate) arteries. Glomerular changes are of four main types:

(1) *Diffuse sclerosis* of the vascular tufts with thickening and hyalinisation of basement membranes and supporting mesangium.

(2) *Nodular lesions* variable in size and number, occurring as hyaline, eosinophilic, often laminated deposits in the mesangium, usually towards the periphery of the vascular tufts—the Kimmelstiel-Wilson lesion.

(3) *Fibrin cap lesions:* located in or around peripheral capillary loops.

(4) *Capsular drop lesions:* similar in appearance to (3) but located below the epithelium of Bowman's capsule. These may be multiple in an individual glomerulus and are regarded by some as specific for this disease. Arterioles show increased hyalinisation.

*Tubular changes:* proximal tubules commonly contain excess lipids and protein; basement membranes are thickened and there may be luminal protein casts.

*The interstitium:* changes vary depending on the degree of ischaemia and incidence of pyelonephritis. The latter may be complicated by necrotising papillitis.

*Clinical effects:* in young subjects, despite adequate treatment, renal complications usually arise after ten to fifteen years as proteinuria; a minority with nodular glomerular lesions proceed to a nephrotic syndrome; hypertension and nitrogen retention are more closely linked to the diffuse glomerular sclerotic lesions. In older, controlled subjects the prognosis is better; renal effects in all groups are adversely modified by pyelonephritis and hypertension.

## Gout

This disease, the result of faulty purine metabolism, may be of primary type or secondary to excessive nuclear breakdown in white cells in leukaemia or in myelo-proliferative disorders.

*Pathological changes* are mainly non-specific. Glomeruli are usually normal; the only specific abnormality is the precipitation of urates as stones within the pelvi-calyx or as crystals within renal tubules sometimes associated with giant cells.

*Clinical effects* depend on the degree of nephron damage and are preceded by many months of hyperuricaemia. There may be early albuminuria and microscopic haematuria or pyuria; later phases reflect progressive renal failure and deterioration of renal function may be hastened by pyelonephritis.

**Fig. 132.** Severe diabetic nephropathy. There is reduction of kidney size and subcapsular cortical surface is pale and granular (*right*). Transverse section of interlobar-arcuate arteries shows severe atherosclerosis (*left*)

**Fig. 133.** Mild diabetic nephropathy. Apart from pallor of some renal medullae there is no significant abnormality

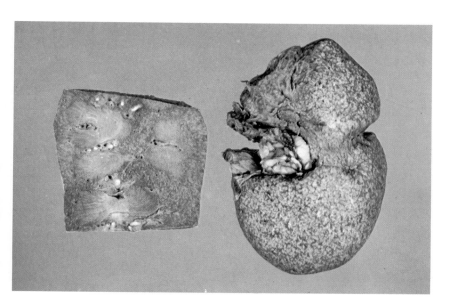

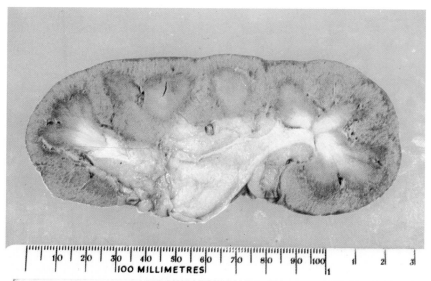

**Fig. 134.** Severe diabetic nephropathy. Diabetic hyaline (red) has infiltrated arteries, arterioles and glomeruli and there is considerable tubular damage (MSB x 80)

**Fig. 135.** Pronounced mesangial thickening as a feature of diabetic glomerulosclerosis (PAS x 352)

**Fig. 136.** Kimmelstiel-Wilson lesions of different ages appear as red or blue nodules in mesangium (MSB x 550)

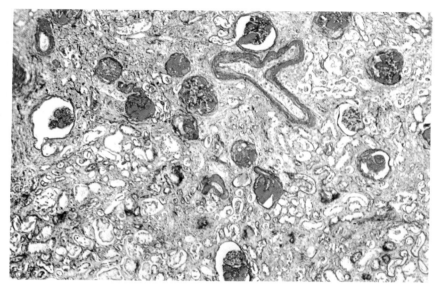

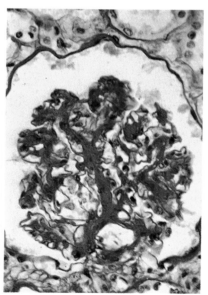
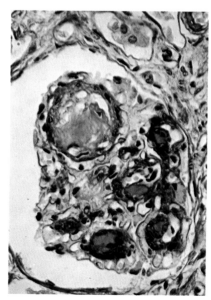

**Fig. 137.** Fibrin cap lesion (red) associated with Kimmelstiel-Wilson nodules (blue) in the glomerulus, and tiny "capsular drops" at centre right. Diabetic hyaline has infiltrated walls of afferent arteriole (MSB x 330)

**Fig. 138.** Capsular drop appears as red deposit at 12 o'clock. The glomerulus is diffusely sclerosed (PAS x 330)

**Fig. 139.** Necrosis of renal papillae (*arrowed*) is occasionally a feature of diabetic nephropathy

**Fig. 140.** Edge of necrotic focus in renal papilla (*bottom left*) with inflammatory infiltration of surrounding tissue (H and E x 132)

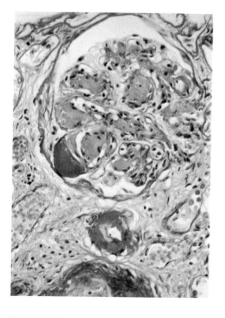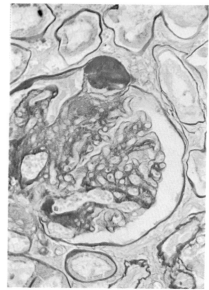

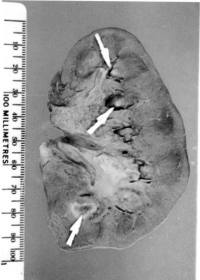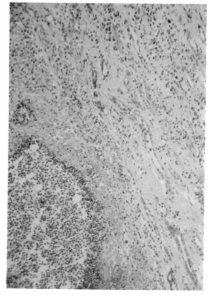

**Fig. 141.** Kidney in gout. Urate crystals in renal tubule with regeneration of damaged epithelium (H and E x 330)

**Fig. 142.** Urate crystals are bi-refringent to polarised light (H and E x 330)

**Fig. 143.** Renal gout. Urate crystals give a positive (grey-green) Schultz reaction (Schultz x 330)

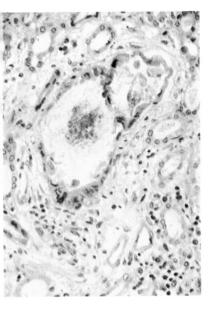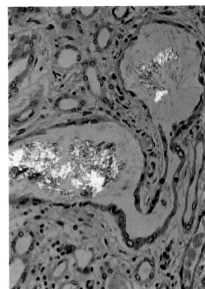

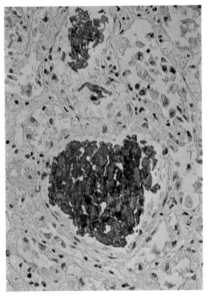

# GROUP II

## *Systemic lupus erythematosus*

*Pathological changes:* The kidneys are involved in about 80 per cent of cases. The damage is mainly glomerular and may take the following forms:
(1) Focal glomerulonephritis, with fibrinoid necrosis of capillary walls.
(2) Hyalin thrombi within capillary loops.
(3) Diffuse basement membrane thickening—the "wire-loop" lesion.
(4) Advanced sclerosis, of lobular or diffuse distribution.
Gross renal changes reflect the stage and form of the disease.

*Clinical effects* vary from mild proteinuria to those of a proliferative glomerulonephritis in an acute, rapidly progressive or chronic form. About a fifth of cases present with a partial (lacking hypercholesterolaemia) or complete, nephrotic syndrome. Active disease is often associated with anti-nuclear factor (A.N.F.) in the serum and L.E. cell formation in response to serum L.E. factor.

The short term prognosis for acute episodes is usually good with resolution of the glomerulitis. For patients with nephrotic syndrome or with evidence of renal failure, the outlook is always poor.


## *Polyarteritis nodosa*

*Pathological changes:* In about 80 per cent of cases, medium arteries, arterioles or glomeruli are involved in a focal necrotising arteritis with infarction as a common complication. Acute lesions comprise fibrinoid necrosis and thrombosis with intense inflammatory cell infiltration. Healed lesions produce vascular scarring with rupture of the elastic lamina and stenosis by organised thrombus or hyperplastic intima. Glomerular lesions may heal to form scars within the tufts.

*Clinical effects:* Patients present with haematuria, proteinuria or as cases of acute proliferative glomerulonephritis. Rarely extensive infarction may cause acute renal failure. Spontaneous or steroid-induced cures or remissions of acute episodes occur, but the outlook in most cases is poor, the later phases being marked by renal failure and hypertension.

## Systemic sclerosis

Renal involvement may occur in either the peripheral (acro-sclerotic) or central rapidly progressive forms of the disease.

*Pathological changes* include basement membrane thickening similar to, but of milder degree than, the "wire-loop" S.L.E. lesions. Fibrinoid necrosis and thrombosis of afferent arterioles usually extends into the glomerular capillaries. Interlobular arteries are narrowed by mucoid intimal hyperplasia and there may be small infarcts and areas of tubular atrophy.

*Clinical effects:* In the chronic form of the disease, renal symptoms may be restricted to proteinuria only. The acute form produces rapid renal failure with hypertension.


## Goodpasture's syndrome

## (Lung purpura and glomerulonephritis)

This rare disease affects mainly young males.

*Pathological changes:* The disease starts as a focal glomerulo-nephritis, progressing rapidly to generalised necrotising glomerulitis with prominent capsular crescents. The glomerular urinary space and the renal tubules often contain red blood cells.

*Clinical effects* comprise lung haemorrhages and a rapidly progressive glomerulonephritis with blood, protein and granular casts in the urine. Remissions of the disease have followed high steroid dosage but the prognosis is poor, death resulting from respiratory or renal failure.

**Fig. 144.** Necrotising glomerulonephritis in Systemic Lupus Erythematosus (S.L.E.) shown as fibrinoid (red) necrosis of capillary loops and focal cellular damage (MSB x 330)

**Fig. 145.** Widespread fibrinoid involvement of glomerular capillaries in S.L.E. (MSB x 330)

**Fig. 146.** S.L.E. showing characteristic "wire-loop" lesion of glomerular capillaries producing a uniform thickening of basement membranes (PAS x 286)

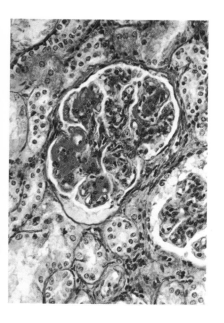

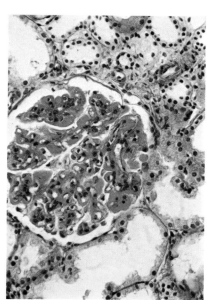

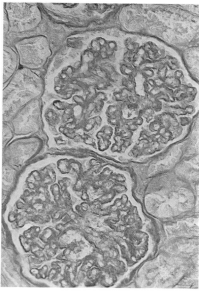

**Fig. 147.** Renal biopsy specimen showing proliferative change and capsular crescents in case of S.L.E. (H and E x 110)

**Fig. 148.** Advanced diffuse glomerular sclerosis in S.L.E. with chronic inflammatory infiltration of intertubular interstitium (PAS x 286)

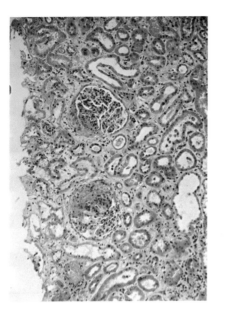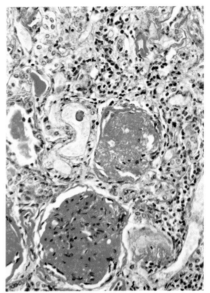

**Fig. 149.** Polyarteritis nodosa (PN) in acute phase. Glomeruli are diffusely hypercellular. Fibrinoid foci are difficult to identify at low magnification (H and E x 55)

**Fig. 150.** Disruption of glomerular structure by proliferative change and fibrinoid necrosis in acute PN (MSB x 330)

**Fig. 151.** Segmental fibrinoid necrosis (red) of interlobular artery in acute PN (MSB x 198)

**Fig. 152.** Transverse section through necrotic focus in interlobular artery showing destruction of vessel wall (red), fibrinoid deposition and inflammatory infiltration (MSB x 330)

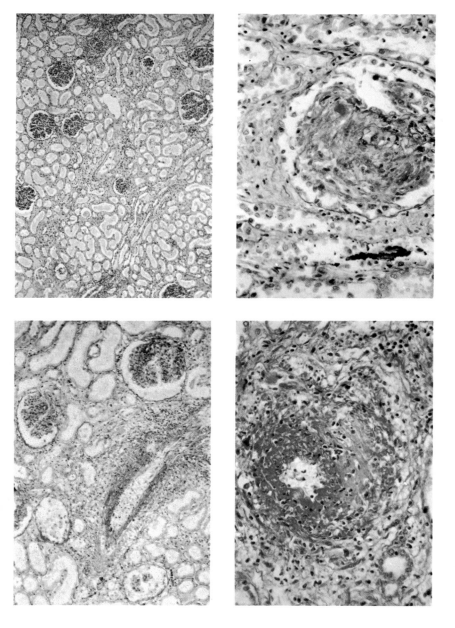

**Fig. 153.** Healed focus of PN in arcuate artery following steroid treatment showing breakdown of elastic fibres and distortion of normal vessel structure (EVG x 165)

**Fig. 154.** Healed focus of PN in arcuate artery showing disruption of internal elastic lamina (in 4–5 o'clock region of circumference) with organised thrombus in arterial lumen (*left*) (MSB x 550)

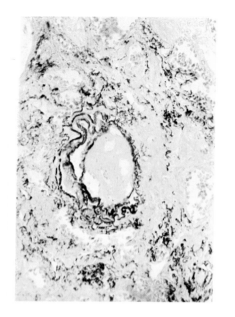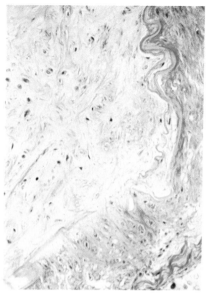

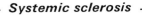
**Fig. 155.** Hemisected kidney in systemic sclerosis (SS) showing normal kidney size, but cortex is diffusely mottled and contains several minute infarcts

**Fig. 156.** Fibrinoid necrosis (red) of afferent arteriole in SS (MSB x 308)

**Fig. 157.** Fibrinoid necrosis extending into glomerular capillaries in SS (MSB x 308)

**Fig. 158.** Transverse section of interlobular artery in SS showing intimal thickening (EVG x 308)

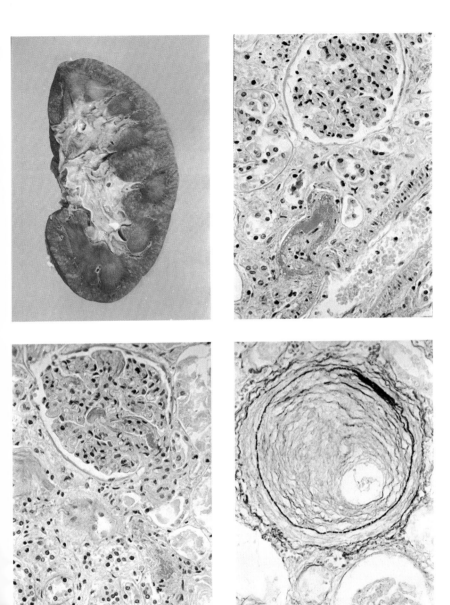

**Fig. 159.** Fulminating acute diffuse glomerulonephritis in Goodpasture's Syndrome (GS) showing fibrinoid necrosis and cell proliferation throughout glomeruli and haemorrhage in some renal tubules (H and E x 66)

**Fig. 160.** Glomeruli from a case of GS showing necrotising inflammation in capillary tufts (H and E x 308)

**Fig. 161.** Case of GS showing mixed necrosis and sclerosis of the destructive glomerular process (H and E x 308)

**Fig. 162.** Lung in GS showing intra alveolar haemorrhage containing (brown) haemosiderin-laden macrophages (MSB x 330)

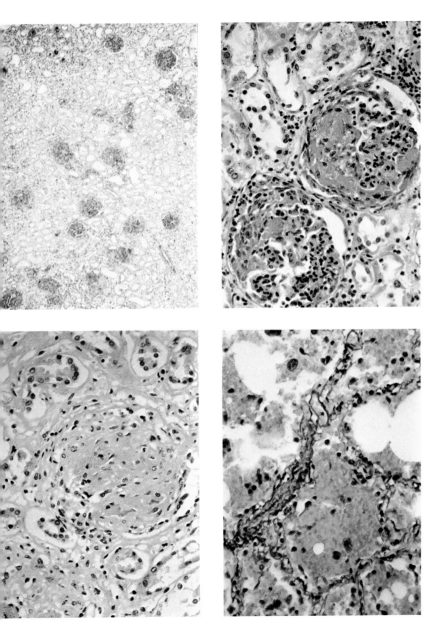

## GROUP III

### Amyloidosis

Amyloid disease may occur as primary, secondary or familial forms. Although all may involve the kidney, secondary amyloidosis usually produces the severest nephropathies.

*Pathological changes* result from the deposition of a largely proteinous, insoluble material in vessels, glomeruli, tubules and interstitial tissues. At the light microscope level, amyloid stains selectively, but non-specifically, with a range of dyes, and electron-optically it comprises both fibrillar and amorphous components.

*Clinical effects* are often mild, relative to the extent of amyloid infiltration. These may be restricted to proteinuria or extend to a full nephrotic syndrome, particularly if complicated (as in a minority of cases) by thrombosis of renal veins. Cases with advanced disease tend to develop hypertension and renal failure. The prognosis is difficult to assess; the renal changes, though irreversible, may allow reasonably good function for several years although few patients survive the onset of oedema by more than eighteen months.

### Myelomatosis

In this disease, abnormal plasma cells secrete abnormal proteins. These appear in the serum as gammaglobulins. Another abnormal protein, of low molecular weight (Bence Jones protein), also appears in the urine of over 50 per cent of cases. It is mainly this latter group which develop renal complications.

*Pathological changes* result mainly from formation of protein casts which obstruct the tubules or provoke a giant cell response within them. Hypercalcaemia from bone involvement by the myeloma cells may cause renal calcification, and a form of "paramyloid" may be formed in the renal vessels and tubules. The glomeruli appear normal or may show thickening of capillary basement membranes.

*Clinical effects* include proteinuria, renal failure—mainly of chronic type—and a tendency to develop pyelonephritis as a result of a lowered resistance to infection. The prognosis is poor, death usually occurring within a few months of renal involvement.

## Waldenström's macroglobulinaemia

In this disease there is a homogeneous increase of IgM in the serum and an abnormal lymphoid cellular response.

*Pathological changes* include deposits of IgM within glomerular capillaries, usually below their endothelial lining. A minority of cases also show amyloid infiltrates.

*Clinical effects* may be limited to proteinuria, or, in advanced cases, may extend to renal failure.

## Sickle cell disease

*Pathological changes* are circulatory and involve both cortex and medulla. Glomerular capillaries are dilated and congested with sickled red cells; infarcts are common in both cortex and medulla.

*Clinical effects:* Haematuria and a loss of ability to concentrate the urine are the main symptoms; development of a nephrotic syndrome has been reported.

## Leukaemia

*Pathological changes* include focal or diffuse leukaemic cell infiltrates within the kidney substance. Platelet deficiency may lead to haemorrhages in the mucosa of the pelvi-calyx, and urates may crystallise in the renal tubules.

*Clinical effects* are usually haematuria or mild proteinuria, occasionally complicated by an obstructive nephropathy if there is significant urate deposition.

**Fig. 163.** Renal amyloidosis. Hemisected kidney from a patient with nephrotic syndrome, showing characteristic wide, pale, cortex

**Fig. 164.** Amyloid infiltration of glomerular capillaries producing thickened basement membranes (Congo Red x 330)

**Fig. 165.** Congo Red stained section examined by polarised light produces a green dichroic effect. This is probably the most specific histological reaction for amyloid (Congo Red x 198)

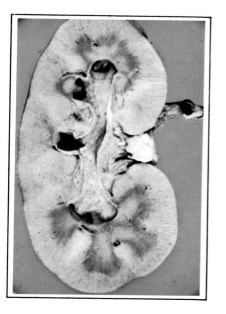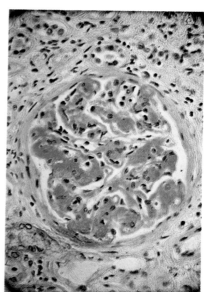

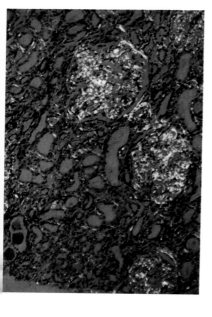

**Fig. 166.** Glomerular amyloid giving yellow fluorescence with thioflavine T under U/V excitation. This is a useful selective but non-specific method for histological demonstration of amyloid (Thioflavine T x 330)

**Fig. 167.** Many amyloids give a metachromatic (red-purple) reaction to rosanilin dyes (Methyl violet x 330)

**Fig. 168.** Amyloid infiltration of tubular basement membranes fluoresces with thioflavine T under U/V excitation. Intra-tubular (protein) casts react only weakly (Thioflavine T x 66)

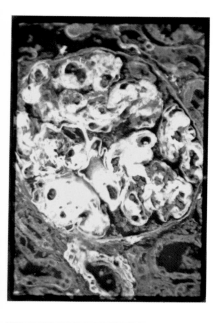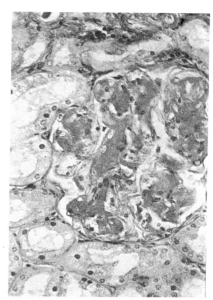

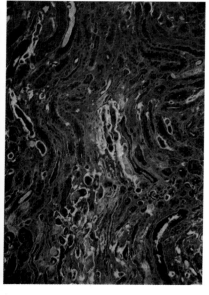

**Fig. 169.** Experimental renal amyloidosis. Early amyloid infiltration induced in glomerulus of a rabbit by repeated casein injection. Electron micrograph showing:
  2—epithelial cell
  3—basement membrane
  14—focus of amyloid infiltration
  15—endothelium
  (x 5500 nm)

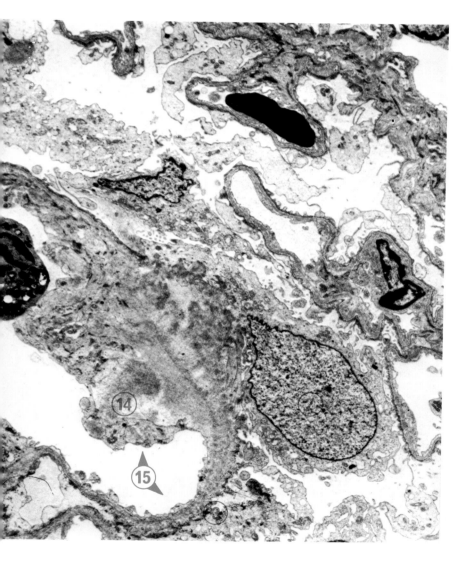

**Fig. 170.** Enlargement of part of Fig. 169 showing fibrillar structure of sub-endothelial amyloid
   3—basement membrane
   15—endothelium
   16—amyloid
   (x  18,700 nm)

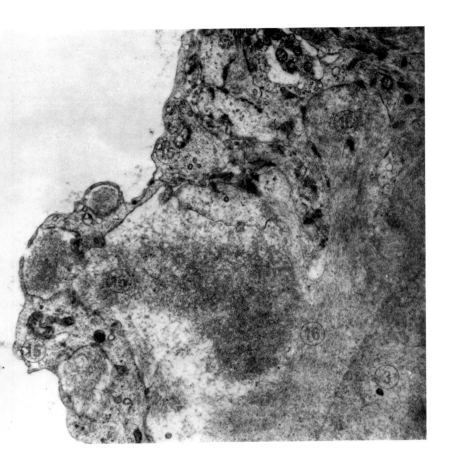

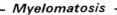

**Fig. 171.** Hemisected kidney in myelomatosis showing swelling and pallor of cortex with diffuse haemorrhages on its subcapsular aspect (about 12 o'clock) and in peripelvic fat

**Fig. 172.** Prominent casts in renal tubules in myelomatosis; these are often associated with giant cell reaction (*top right*) (MSB x 330)

**Fig. 173.** Calcification (*top left*) of tubular casts and severe tubular disruption in myelomatosis (MSB x 330)

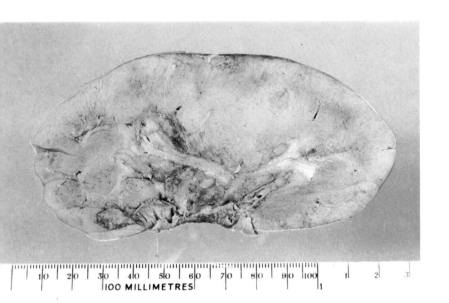

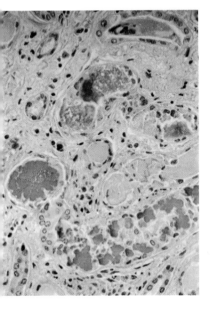
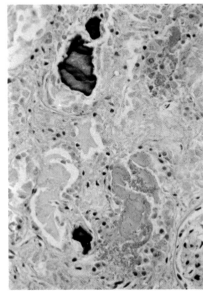

**Fig. 174.** Rarely crystals of abnormal myeloma protein occur in renal tubules. These appear as eosinophilic, weakly refractile, rods or prisms (H and E x 330)

**Fig. 175.** Bone marrow from patient whose kidney is shown in Fig. 171, showing replacement of normal marrow by neoplastic plasma cells (H and E x 550)

## Waldenström's macroglobulinaemia

**Fig. 176.** The subcapsular cortex shows a zone of dense cell infiltration in macroglobulinaemia (H and E x 55)

**Fig. 177.** The cortical cell infiltrates (Fig. 176) are mainly of small lymphocytes —occasional forms resemble small plasma cells (PAS x 550)

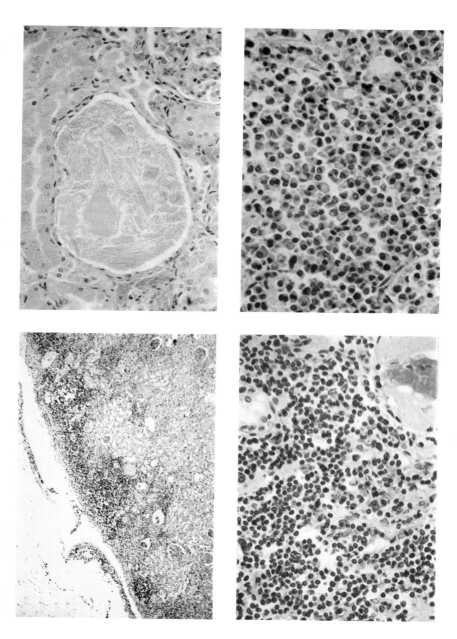

**Fig. 178.** Sickle cell disease showing generalised intense red cell engorgement of glomerular capillary systems (H and E x 224)

**Fig. 179.** Higher magnification of one of the glomeruli shown in Fig. 178; sickled red cells can be seen in capillary lumina (H and E x 800)

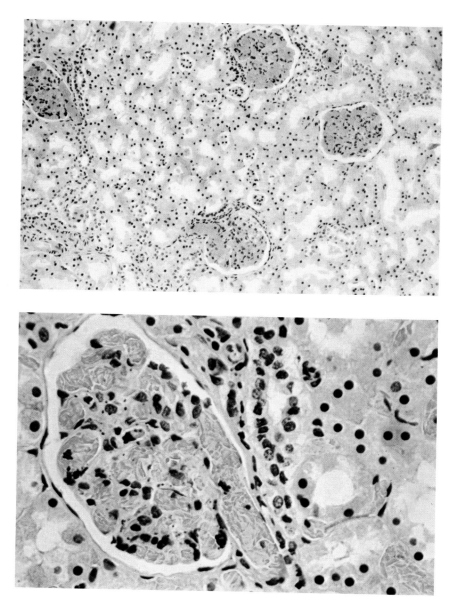

**Fig. 180.** Hemisected kidney from a male aged 50 with acute lymphoblastic leukaemia. Note pallor of the parenchyma and haematoma formation in pelvi-calyx

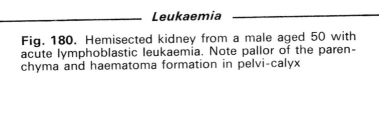

**Fig. 181.** Section from edge of haematoma shown in Fig. 180; the calyceal mucosa is infiltrated with leukaemic cells (H and E x 480)

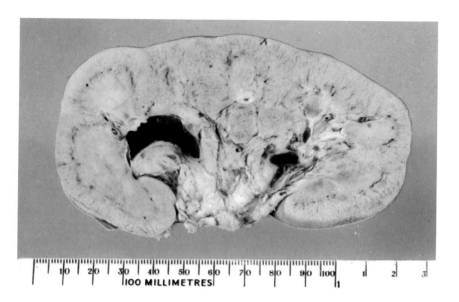

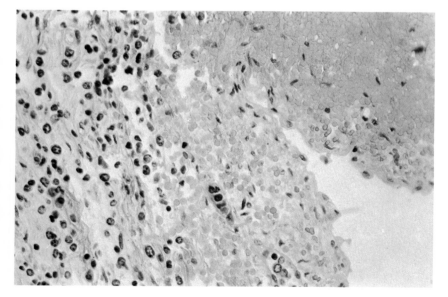

# Tubular Diseases

## Degenerations

Various so-called "degenerative" changes may affect the renal tubular epithelium (mainly of the proximal convolutions), but few of them have a specific cause.

*Hydropic degeneration* is seen as a fine stippling of the epithelial cell cytoplasm and may follow dextran infusion, although it also occurs in a wide range of clinical disorders. *Potassium deficiency* which may complicate chronic intestinal disease or diabetes mellitus produces a coarser cell vacuolation.

*Hyaline degeneration* of proximal tubule cells commonly accompanies proteinuria; it produces a fairly coarse cytoplasmic granularity indicative of increased lysosomal activity. *Fatty droplets* are common in diabetic kidneys or in renal lesions associated with the nephrotic syndrome.

## Acute tubular necrosis

This is one of the more common and important causes of acute renal failure. Two mechanisms contribute to its production:

   (a) toxic damage to the sensitive renal tubular epithelium, and
   (b) ischaemic damage to tubular basement membranes; both may operate simultaneously.

Toxic changes may be produced by chemicals, e.g., mercury salts, ethylene glycol, etc., mainly to the proximal convolutions; ischaemic damage following severe shock as in crush or burn injuries, haemorrhage or infections, primarily involves the distal convolutions.

The extent of the inflammatory changes in and around damaged tubules and the composition of the lower nephron casts vary with the cause. The outcome depends on the severity of the damage. Intact tubular basement membranes allow for regeneration of their lining epithelium and functional restoration from the clinical oliguria or anuria and increasing azotaemia which mark the early phases. The proportion of patients who recover nowadays is significantly higher than formerly, but the prognosis varies with the cause.

**Fig. 182.** Hydropic degeneration of proximal tubules in a patient dying with congestive heart failure. The tubular epithelium is swollen and finely granular (H and E x 330)

**Fig. 183.** Severe degree of hydropic degeneration in proximal tubules in a patient infused with dextran following burn injuries (PAS x 363)

**Fig. 184.** Hyaline degeneration of proximal tubular epithelium appearing as coarse, red, intracytoplasmic granules (MSB x 330)

**Fig. 185.** Hyaline degeneration. In this case the granules appear in varying concentrations in epithelium of proximal tubules (H and E x 330)

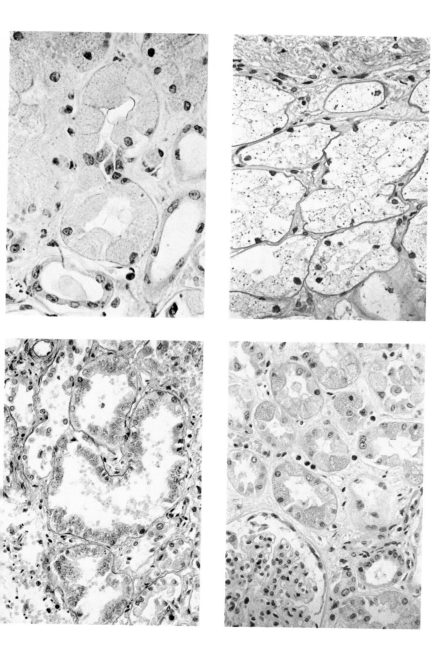

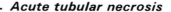

**Fig. 186.** Acute tubular necrosis as a result of surgical shock. Hemisected kidneys showing pallor and swelling of their cortices and congested medullae. Kidney on right also has a very recent renal artery thrombosis

**Fig. 187.** Severe damage to distal convoluted tubules in "boundary zone", and early inflammatory cell infiltration in a case of acute tubular necrosis following multiple injuries (H and E x 66)

**Fig. 188.** Dilated proximal tubules with evidence of tubular epithelial regeneration; from specimen shown in Fig. 186 (H and E x 330)

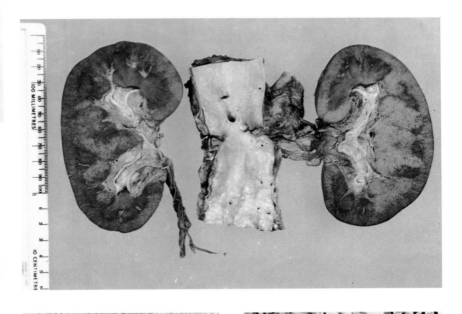

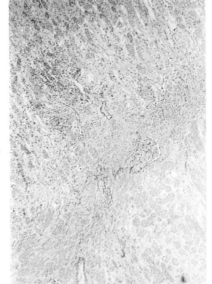

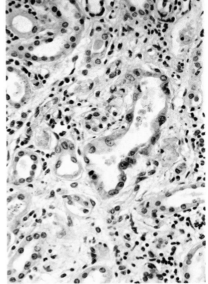

**Fig. 189.** Tubulorhexis in acute tubular necrosis. There is an interstitial inflammatory infiltration around the focus of tubular rupture (H and E x 220)

**Fig. 190.** Pigment casts in collecting tubules in a case of acute tubular necrosis (H and E x 132)

**Fig. 191.** Nucleated cells (? haemopoiesis) in vasa recta of a patient surviving six days after severe shock from multiple injuries (MSB x 297)

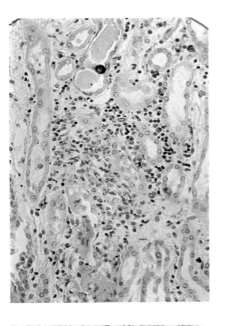

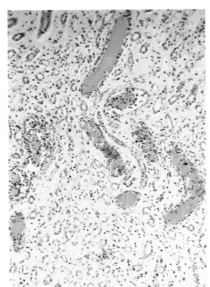

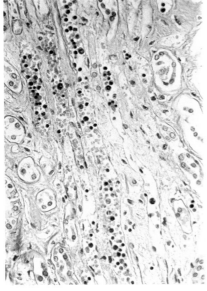

# Renal Stones and Calcification

## Renal stones

Renal stones comprise solid matter (usually inorganic salts) precipitated from solution in the kidney tubules or pelvi-calyx. Calcium phosphates alone or in combination with oxalates are the most common, but uric acid, urates and carbonates, and to a lesser extent, cystine, leucine, xanthine and other amino-acids or purines may also contribute. Calcification of the renal papillae (Randall's plaques) with subsequent sloughing into the kidney calyx may form the nucleus for some stone formations. Calcium and cystine stones are radio-opaque; non-opaque stones (e.g., uric acid) may be identified by pyelography.

The clinical effects vary widely; there may be none or there may be spasmodic pain and haematuria, urinary obstructive symptoms or repeated bouts of complicating infection.

## Renal calcification and the parathyroid glands

Increased levels of urinary calcium (usually reflecting increased serum calcium levels) promote calcification or stone formation. Most often this results from *primary hyperparathyroidism*—a condition in which tumours of the parathyroid glands (usually solitary adenomas) or diffuse hyperplasia produce excess parathormone which mobilises skeletal calcium.

Hypercalcaemia may also result from sarcoidosis, invasion of the skeleton by metastatic tumours, myelomatosis, prolonged immobilisation or, in rare instances, from excessive intake of vitamin D, or milk-alkali mixtures by peptic ulcer patients.

Calcium deposition occurs mainly in the tubular basement membranes and cells and to a lesser extent in the renal arterial system.

*Renal osteodystrophy:* A proportion of patients with chronic renal failure due to primary renal disease develop abnormalities of bone structure and mineralisation along with lowered or normal levels of ionic serum calcium and variable elevations of serum phosphorus. Associated with this biochemical abnormality there is enlargement of the parathyroid glands—resulting in the condition of *secondary hyperparathyroidism*. The kidneys are nearly always small and fibrotic—examples of so-called "end-stage kidneys" in which it is rarely possible to define the primary renal disorder and in which the degree of calcification varies greatly.

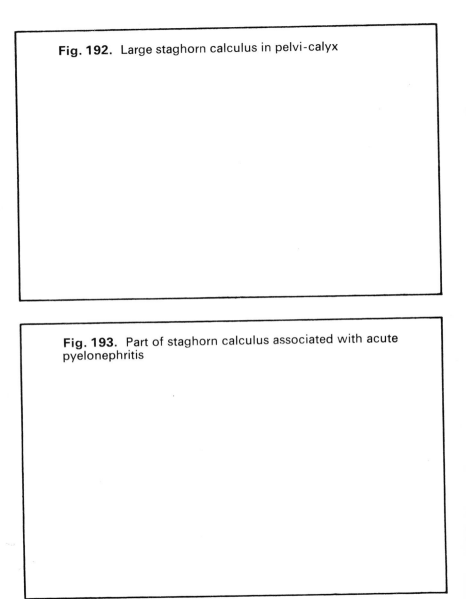

**Fig. 192.** Large staghorn calculus in pelvi-calyx

**Fig. 193.** Part of staghorn calculus associated with acute pyelonephritis

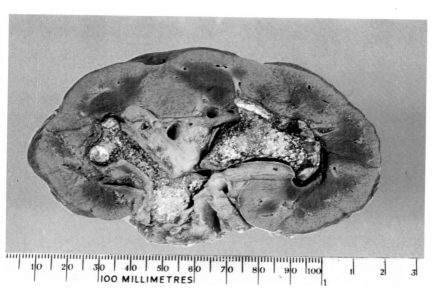

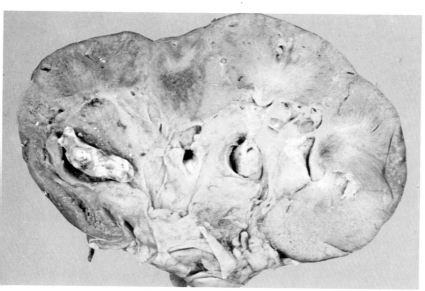

**Fig. 194.** Radiograph showing large staghorn calculus in right kidney

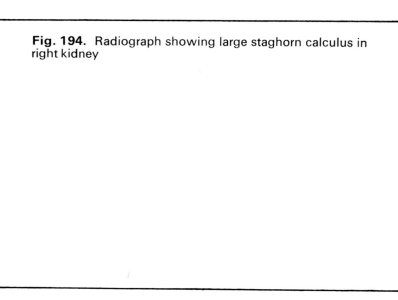

**Fig. 195.** Calculus formation in kidneys (more pronounced in right) of patient with medullary sponge kidney. This is a common form of presentation of this renal malformation

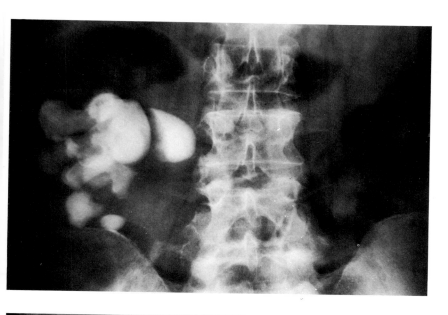
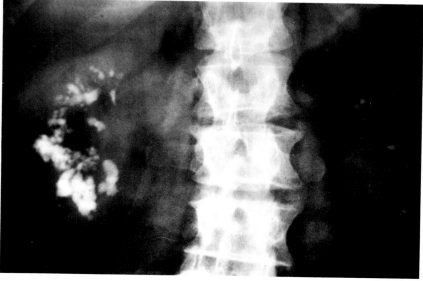

**Fig. 196.** Solitary mixed stone of mulberry appearance in renal pelvis

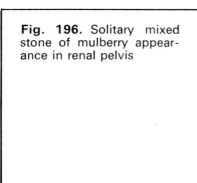

**Fig. 197.** Enlargement (x 7) of stone removed from specimen in Fig. 196

**Fig. 198.** Fragments of mixed stone polarised to show crystal lattice of fracture surfaces (x 66)

**Fig. 199.** Numerous oxalate crystals in kidney tubules examined under partially crossed polaroids (MSB x 66)

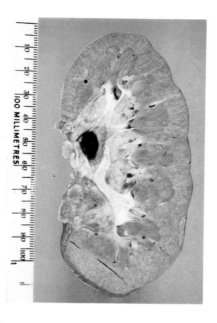
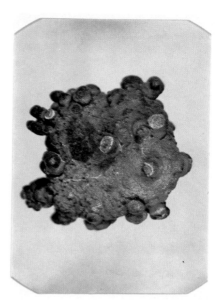
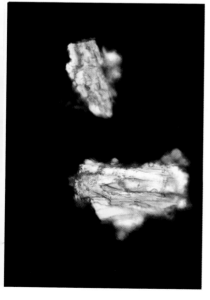
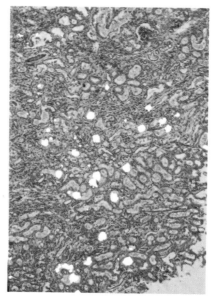

**Fig. 200.** Leucine-type crystals (polarised) in renal tubules of patient with liver failure (H and E x 330)

**Fig. 201.** Primary hyperparathyroidism. Parathyroid adenoma of uniform chief cell type (H and E x 88)

**Fig. 202.** Bone from case shown in Fig. 201, showing the changes of osteitis fibrosa with prominent osteoclastic proliferation (H and E x 88)

**Fig. 203.** Kidney from case illustrated in Fig. 201 showing focal calcification in and around renal tubules (H and E x 88)

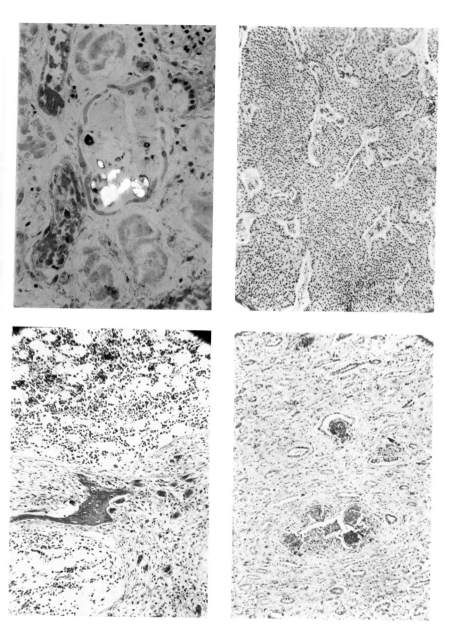

**Fig. 204.** Secondary hyperparathyroidism. The patient died of renal failure due to slowly progressive glomerulonephritis as reflected in both kidneys. The specimen on the left shows the enlarged pale parathyroid glands lying between the oesophagus and thyroid lobes

**Fig. 205.** Kidneys, ureters, and urinary bladder from patient with secondary parathyroid hyperplasia. There is advanced renal destruction due to bilateral chronic pyelonephritis and pyonephrosis

**Fig. 206.** Hyperplastic parathyroid gland from case illustrated in Fig. 205 showing both chief cell and oxyntic cell (*centre*) forms (H and E x 330)

**Fig. 207.** Bone section from patient concerned in Fig. 205 showing active osteoclasis and fibrosis as features of renal osteodystrophy (H and E x 550)

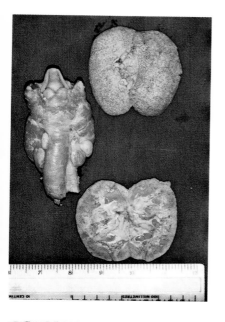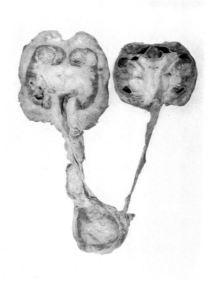

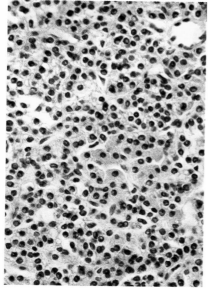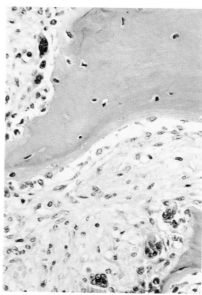

**Fig. 208.** Extensive renal calcification (mainly of the medulla) occurring in association with bronchogenic carcinoma (see Fig. 210)

**Fig. 209.** Tissue from renal medulla of kidney illustrated in Fig. 208 showing extensive black deposits of calcium (phosphate) (Von Kossa x 198)

**Fig. 210.** Bronchogenic (squamous) carcinoma from patient concerned in Fig. 208. Malignant squamous cells lie above the bronchial cartilage (H and E x 550)

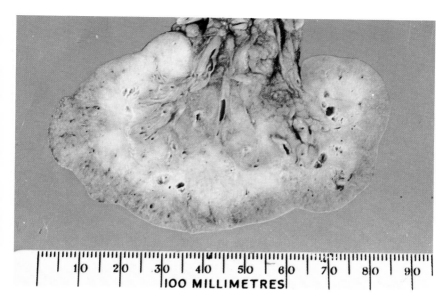

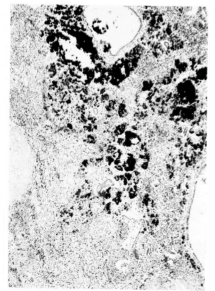
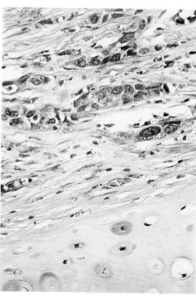

# Hydronephrosis

IN HYDRONEPHROSIS there is dilatation of the renal pelvis and calyces with atrophy of the surrounding kidney tissue. It develops in conditions of chronic or intermittent urinary obstruction either as the result of congenital structural abnormalities or of acquired conditions such as calculus, tumours, enlargement of the prostate or pregnancy. Hydronephrosis may affect one or both kidneys and it varies in severity.

The renal papillae atrophy and the underlying renal lobes become hollowed out, leaving only a rim of tissue beneath a thickened capsule. In early cases, structural changes are minimal, but in long-standing disease, tubular atrophy may be severe with sclerosis of glomeruli and interstitial fibrosis.

The clinical effects vary. If unilateral, hydronephrosis may be symptomless or it may present with haematuria, hypertension or as pyelonephritis when secondarily infected. These symptoms may be augmented by evidence of renal failure if both kidneys are involved. The prognosis relates mainly to the underlying cause.

**Fig. 211.** Hydronephrosis resulting from obstruction of proximal ureter by carcinoma. There is marked atrophy of kidney parenchyma and pelvi-calyceal distension

**Fig. 212.** Transitional cell carcinoma from ureter shown in specimen illustrated in Fig. 211 (H and E x 198)

**Fig. 213.** Severe degree of bilateral hydronephrosis and hydroureter caused by impacted ureteric calculi

**Fig. 214.** Hydroureter and hydronephrosis of left kidney due to ureteric obstruction by carcinoma of urinary bladder

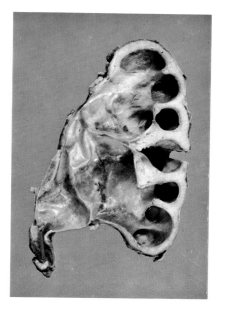
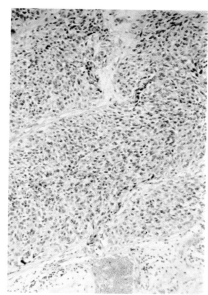
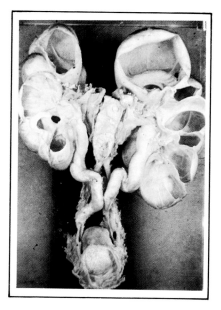
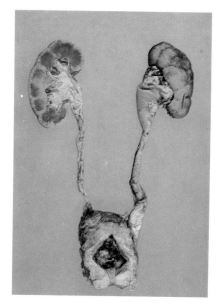

**Fig. 215.** Severe hydronephrosis (*left*) and nephrosclerosis (*right*) in a patient with renal hypertension. The hydronephrosis resulted from pressure by an aberrant renal artery on the pelvi-ureteric junction

**Fig. 216.** Hydronephrosis and excessive peri-pelvic fat in a kidney with multiple calculi, some of which remain in a lesser calyx (*centre right*)

**Fig. 217.** Atrophy of nephrons and glomerular sclerosis account for loss of renal parenchyma in severe hydronephrosis. Section taken from specimen shown in Fig. 211 (MSB x 66)

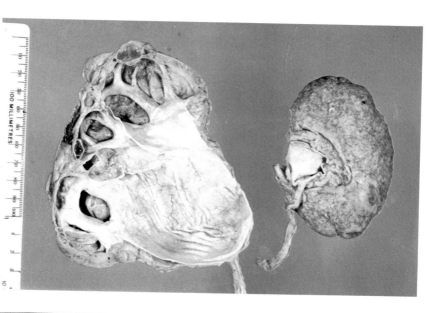

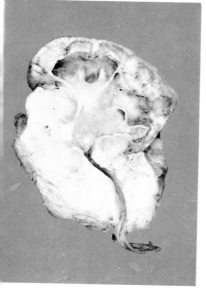

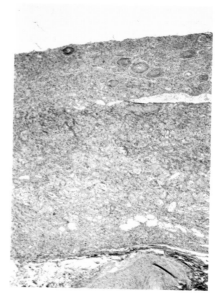

# Renal Neoplasms

TUMOURS in the kidney may be of primary or secondary origin. Primary tumours may be benign or malignant.

## Primary benign tumours

The most common is a cortical tubular adenoma, usually small, solid or cystic and often multiple. Fibromas are more common in the medulla. Rarer tumours include haemangioma, angiolipoma and lipoma. Benign neoplasms are of minor clinical significance, often symptomless and discovered incidentally at autopsy.

## Primary malignant tumours

(1) The most important (though of low incidence in terms of total body tumours) is a tubular carcinoma (Grawitz tumour or hypernephroma). It forms a yellow, often circumscribed, cortical mass with haemorrhagic and necrotic areas, and consists of rather characteristic large, clear or granular cells or, rarely, of spindle cell forms. Clinically it produces painless haematuria, and has a distinctive angiographic vascular pattern. It is only moderately aggressive but tends to invade the renal veins and thus spread to the lungs and other organs.

(2) Wilms' tumour, or nephroblastoma, occurs almost always in young children in whom it represents one of the principal malignancies. It forms an expanding mass of solid, grey tissue with haemorrhagic and cystic areas; histologically it consists of spindle cell masses mixed with primitive glomerular and tubular structures and variable amounts of striped muscle which assume more prominence after radiotherapy. This tumour may be symptomless and present purely as a space-occupying mass, although occasionally it causes haematuria. It is an aggressive tumour, spreads freely and has a poor prognosis.

(3) Tumours of the renal pelvis are mainly of epithelial origin forming papillary or flat growths which frequently ulcerate. Papillary tumours may be multiple, and mainly of transitional cell type with a wide range of differentiation best regarded as representing a continuous spectrum of malignancy. Some of the flat tumours are squamous cell cancers and, in common with all malignancies arising in the kidney pelvis, have a bad prognosis.

## Secondary (metastatic) tumours

Many forms occur, spreading to the kidney by direct extension or via the blood or lymph streams from primary cancers in the bronchus, uterus, breast or other organs, or as part of a dissemination of malignant melanomas or lymphomas.

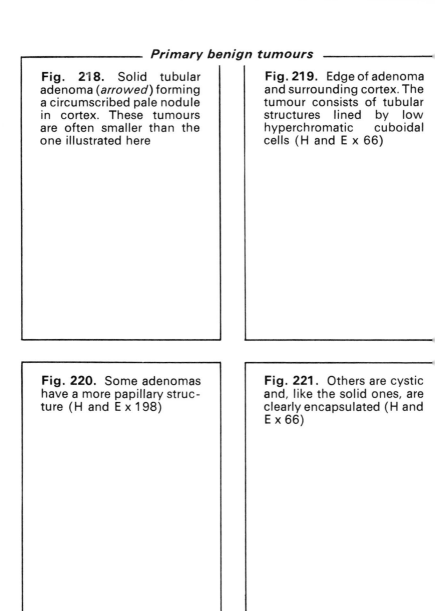

**Fig. 218.** Solid tubular adenoma (*arrowed*) forming a circumscribed pale nodule in cortex. These tumours are often smaller than the one illustrated here

**Fig. 219.** Edge of adenoma and surrounding cortex. The tumour consists of tubular structures lined by low hyperchromatic cuboidal cells (H and E x 66)

**Fig. 220.** Some adenomas have a more papillary struc- ture (H and E x 198)

**Fig. 221.** Others are cystic and, like the solid ones, are clearly encapsulated (H and E x 66)

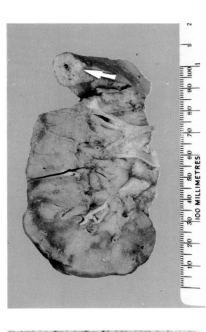

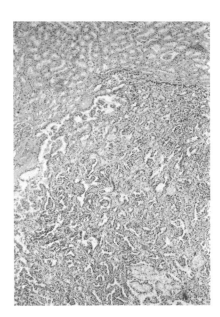

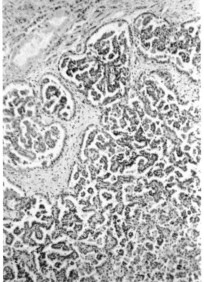

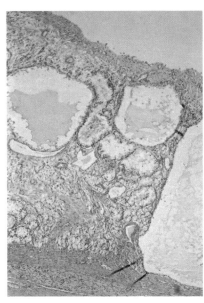

**Fig. 222.** Renal angio-lipoma. This is a rare form of benign tumour consisting of fibro-fatty tissue of varying cellularity and numerous primitive blood vessels (H and E x 66)

**Fig. 223.** Higher magnification of fibro-fatty tissue (*below*) and blood vessels (*above*) from tumour illustrated in Fig. 222 (H and E x 330)

**Fig. 224.** Renal leiomyoma, a benign tumour of smooth muscle origin consists of interlacing muscle bundles (purple), and vascular channels (Acid picro —Mallory x 330)

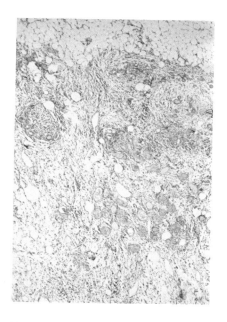 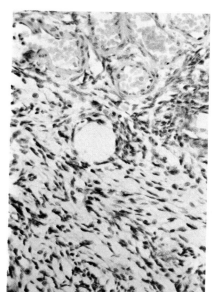

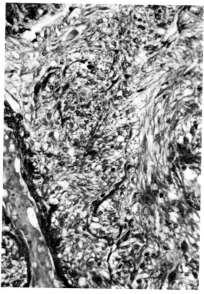

**Fig. 225.** Tubular carcinoma (hypernephroma) forming a spherical mass projecting from upper pole of the kidney

**Fig. 226.** Tubular carcinoma showing extensive haemorrhagic necrosis

**Fig. 227.** Most tubular carcinomas are comprised of large clear or granular cells (H and E x 220)

**Fig. 228.** Higher magnification showing occasional giant tumour cells in tubular carcinoma (H and E x 550)

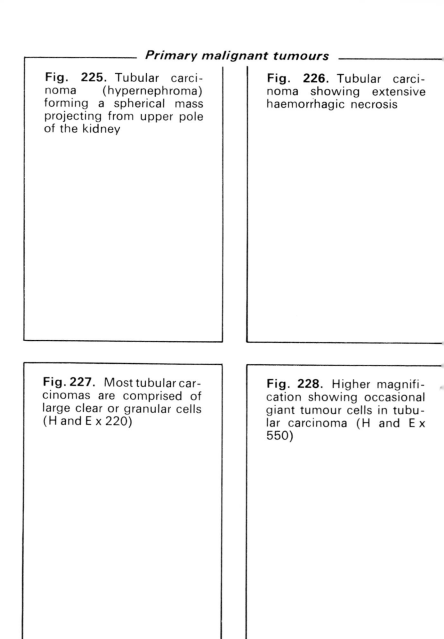

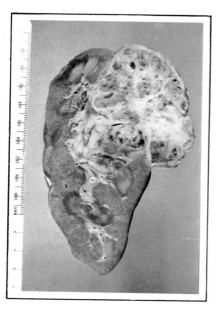

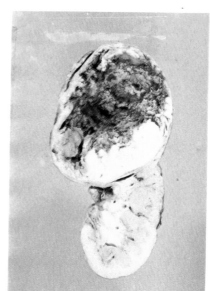

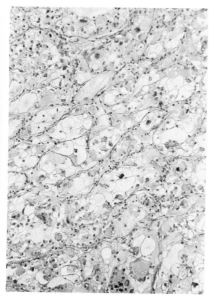

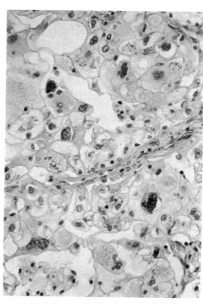

**Fig. 229.** Tubular carcinoma growing into renal pelvis and surrounded by haematoma

**Fig. 230.** Oblique section of kidney involved with a tubular carcinoma which has invaded the renal veins causing them to thrombose (*arrowed*)

**Fig. 231.** Section of renal vein from preceding specimen (Fig. 230). The vein lumen (*above*) is occupied by thrombus (*right*) and tumour (*left*) (MSB x 66)

**Fig. 232.** A less common histological pattern of tubular carcinoma is a spindle cell type. In this case most of the tumour consisted of this form (MSB x 330)

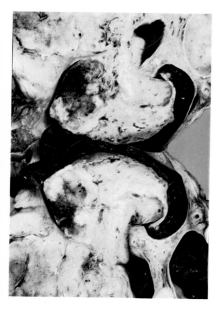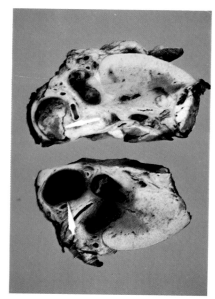

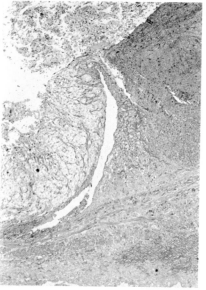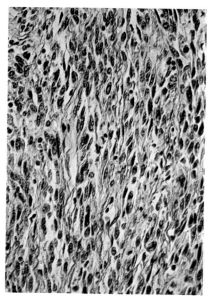

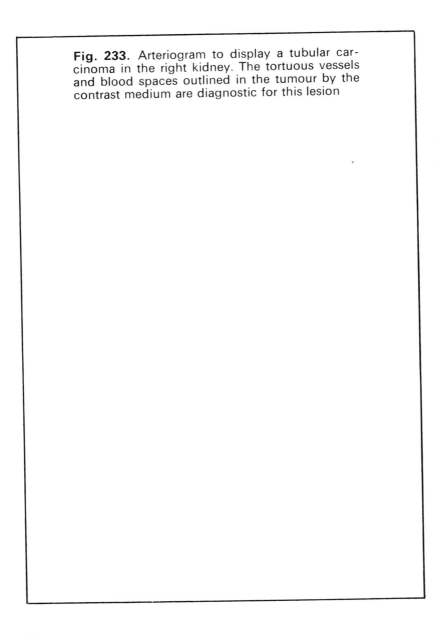

**Fig. 233.** Arteriogram to display a tubular carcinoma in the right kidney. The tortuous vessels and blood spaces outlined in the tumour by the contrast medium are diagnostic for this lesion

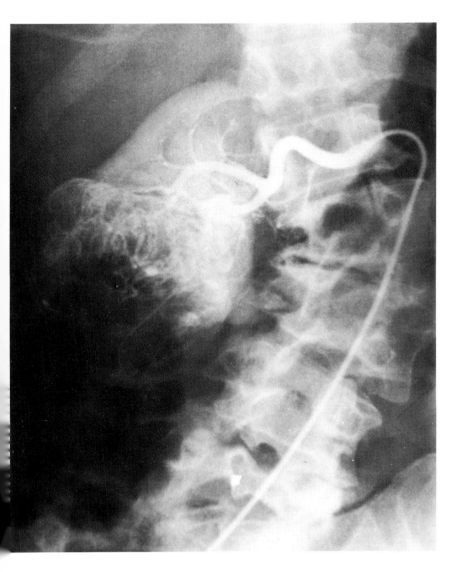

**Fig. 234.** Malignant renal tumour of uncertain histogenesis replacing most of one kidney of a 62-year-old female. The tumour was uniformly white and firm

**Fig. 235.** Histological examination of specimen in Fig. 234 disclosed a uniformly cellular tumour resembling a pericytoma (H and E x 330)

**Fig. 236.** The malignant nature of this lesion (Fig. 234) was confirmed by its spread to the lungs (H and E x 330)

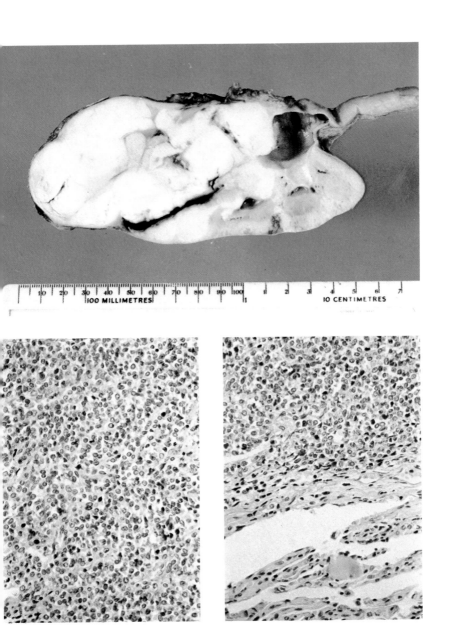

**Fig. 237.** Wilms' tumour or nephroblastoma. The tumour consists of tubular and spindle cell components (H and E x 330)

**Fig. 238.** Following radiotherapy with reduction of epithelial component, muscle fibres become prominent in the tumour (H and E x 220)

**Fig. 239.** Papilloma of renal pelvis showing papillary processes projecting from underlying mucosal membrane (H and E x 2)

**Fig. 240.** The tumour papillae consist of fibrous cores (*lower left*) supporting a multi-layered transitional epithelium. Such tumours have a poorer prognosis than their rather benign appearances would indicate (H and E x 363)

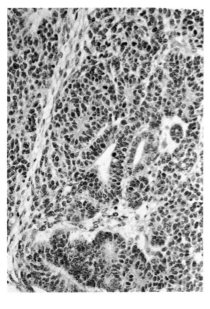
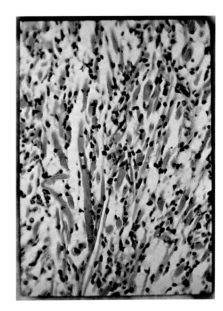
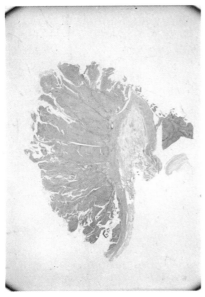
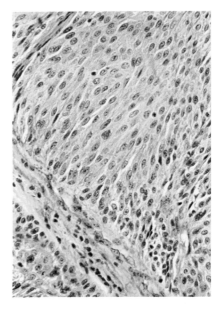

**Fig. 241.** Carcinoma of renal pelvis. The tumour occupies much of the pelvis and has grown out into the pelvic calyces. An internal hydronephrosis has followed

**Fig. 242.** Section from preceding specimen (Fig. 241) showing nuclear pleomorphism of transitional epithelium indicating malignancy (H and E x 330)

**Fig. 243.** Transitional cell carcinoma of renal pelvis showing focus of tumour giant cells (H and E x 550)

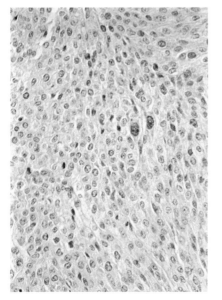

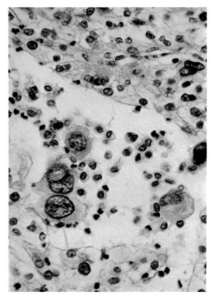

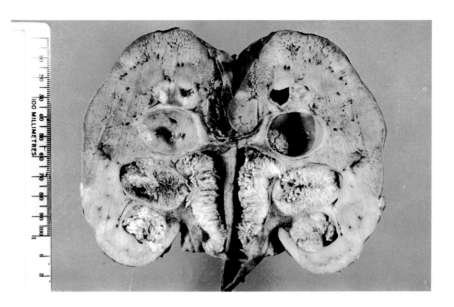

**Fig. 244.** Squamous carcinoma of renal pelvis arising in a patient with renal calculi. The mucosal surface shows malignant change of metaplastic epithelium and invasion of underlying pelvic wall (H and E x 154)

**Fig. 245.** Squamous carcinoma of renal pelvis showing keratinisation of cell nest (*below*) and invasive tumour cells (*above*) (H and E x 352)

**Fig. 246.** Myosarcoma of kidney from female aged 24 years with long history of slowly growing abdominal mass which replaced entire kidney. This rare tumour may represent a form of Wilms' tumour

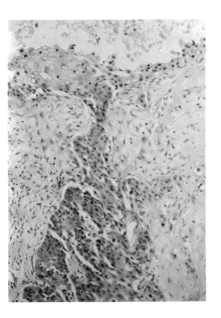
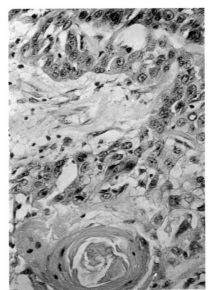
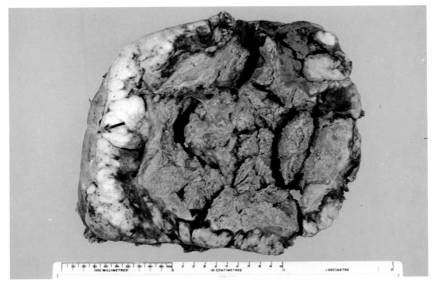

**Fig. 247.** The tumour (Fig. 246) consists of uniform masses of spindle cells (H and E x 66)

**Fig. 248.** Areas of the tumour (Fig. 246) contain giant cell forms (H and E x 352)

## Secondary (metastatic) tumours

**Fig. 249.** Tumour microembolus in kidney glomerulus from primary carcinoma of pancreas. Most of the glomerulus has been replaced by tumour cells (H and E x 330)

**Fig. 250.** Multiple renal metastases from a primary rectal carcinoma. Tumour appears as multiple white nodules on subcapsular surface (*below*) and in kidney parenchyma (*above*)

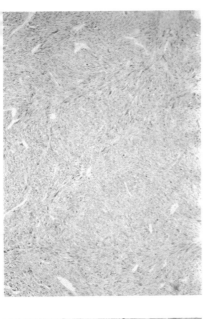

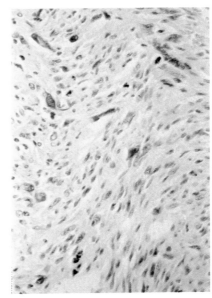

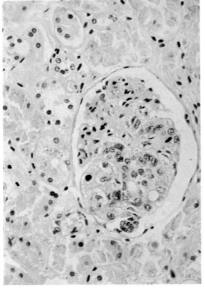

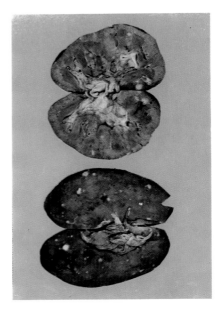

**Fig. 251.** The adeno-carcinomatous nature of the metastases shown in Fig. 250 is confirmed histologically (H and E x 198)

**Fig. 252.** Portion of kidney showing solitary pale metastasis from a primary carcinoma of breast

**Fig. 253.** The histology of the lesion in Fig. 252 confirms its mammary origin (H and E x 352)

**Fig. 254.** Renal involvement in lymphosarcoma; the tissue around the glomerular corpuscle consists mainly of tumour lymphocytes (H and E x 198)

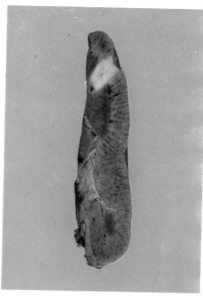

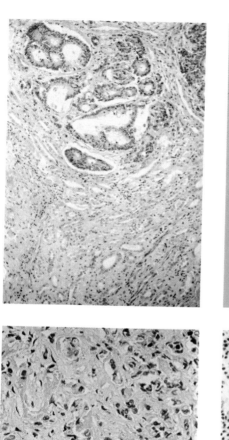

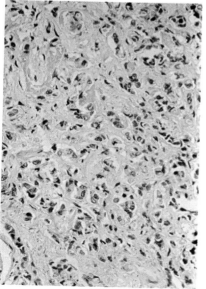

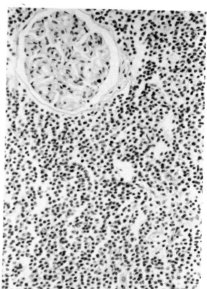

**Fig. 255.** Renal involvement in Hodgkin's disease; there is extensive infiltration of cortex by neoplastic tissue (H and E x 66)

**Fig. 256.** Higher magnification of tumour tissue from Fig. 255 showing the pleomorphic nature of the infiltrate in Hodgkin's disease (H and E x 352)

**Fig. 257.** Renal involvement in acute lymphoblastic leukaemia in female aged 52 years. The most prominent evidence of this disease in gross specimens is haemorrhage into kidney substance and the pelvi-calyx (*cf*. Fig. 180)

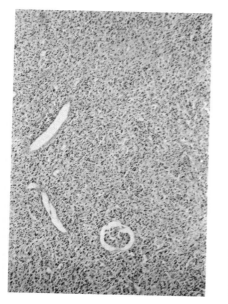

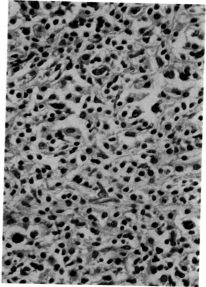

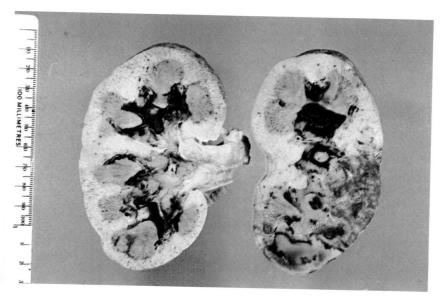

# Renal Transplantation

KIDNEY transplantation has emerged from the experimental stage and now has an established role in the treatment of patients with irreversible renal failure. Transplantation implies a donor source—usually a cadaver, occasionally a blood relative—and a recipient, and the task of successful transfer requires considerable laboratory and clinical skills.

Transplantation of tissue from one individual to another in normal circumstances produces a tissue reaction in the recipient directed at the rejection of the grafted tissue. This is due to presence of histocompatibility (H) antigens on the surfaces of the graft tissue cells which are "foreign" to the recipient. The closer the similarity between the donor and the recipient's tissues in terms of H antigens, the greater the likelihood of a successful transplant. Serological tests to determine these H antigens, referred to as "tissue typing", are therefore an essential preliminary to renal transplantation. In man, as in animals, these H antigens are genetically determined and include the ABO red blood cell antigens and those of the HL-A system which are present on tissue cells of most organs (including the kidney) and of which there are upwards of twenty in number. In view of this complex biological situation it is hardly surprising that a significant proportion of transplanted kidneys are rejected.

## TRANSPLANT REJECTION

### First-set rejection
The tissue reactions which mark the rejection process depend on whether the transplant in question is the first to be grafted to the recipient. If so the process is referred to as a *first-set rejection* which is characterised by lymphoid and plasma cell infiltration in and around the peri-tubular capillaries which break down with escape of fluid and cells into the interstitial tissues. This is followed by damage to proximal tubules, increasing tissue oedema and, in some cases, by fibrinoid necrosis and thrombosis of arteries and arterioles. If the rejection episode is suppressed by therapy, the vessel lesions may heal leaving intimal hyperplasia and ruptures of the internal elastic lamina.

## Second-set rejection

This refers to the rejection of a second or subsequent transplant. The process is more rapid and violent on account of the hypersensitive state of the recipient. The rejected kidney is dull red in colour, the glomeruli are packed with clumped red cells and infarction of the cortex and interstitial haemorrhages rapidly follow, producing anuria within a few hours.

Clinically, rejection is marked by anuria (total failure to secrete urine). This is of rapid onset in second-set rejections in hypersensitive subjects, but it can also result from surgical technical failure. Tubular damage may also result if there is undue delay in transplantation after death of the donor.

The prognosis in renal transplantation is unpredictable in view of the large number of variables involved, not least the genetic compatibilities between donor and recipient. When these are limited to one antigen or less, a large majority of transplants will function well for a few years, and with improvements in tissue-typing and in immunosuppression this period will undoubtedly be increased in the future.

In the section following, Figs. 258–263 apply to "first-set" type rejection; Figs. 264–267 apply to "second-set" rejection in sensitised patients.

**Fig. 258.** First set rejection after 9 weeks' transplantation. The later vascular changes have led to numerous cortical infarcts

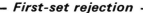

**Fig. 259.** Rejection reaction 4 months after transplantation, showing dense lymphocytic infiltration of the cortex (MSB x 66)

**Fig. 260.** Many of the cells of the interstitial infiltrate demonstrate pyroninophilia (red) of their cytoplasm (Methyl green—pyronin x 330)

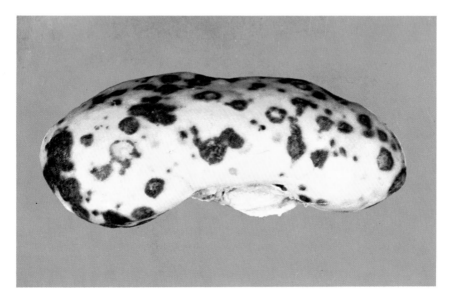

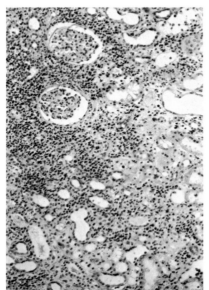
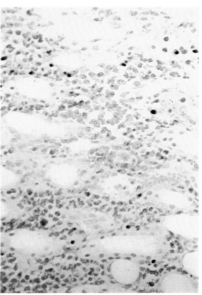

**Fig. 261.** Muscular arteries are occluded by thrombi and intimal hyperplasia (EVG x 240)

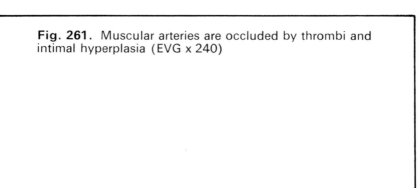

**Fig. 262.** Previous episodes of rejection (treated by immunosuppression therapy) produce focal ruptures of the internal elastic lamina and intimal hyperplasia in muscular arteries (EVG x 240)

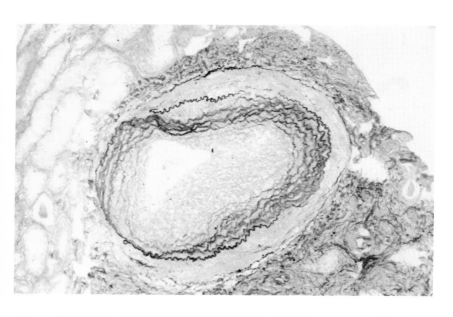

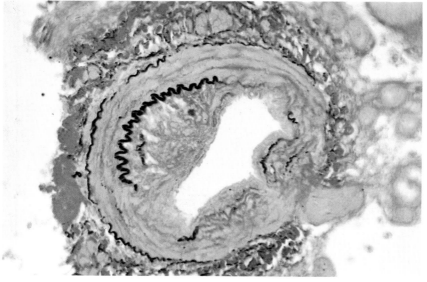

**Fig. 263.** Arteriogram of transplanted kidney undergoing rejection shows failure of contrast medium to penetrate obstructed intra-renal vessels

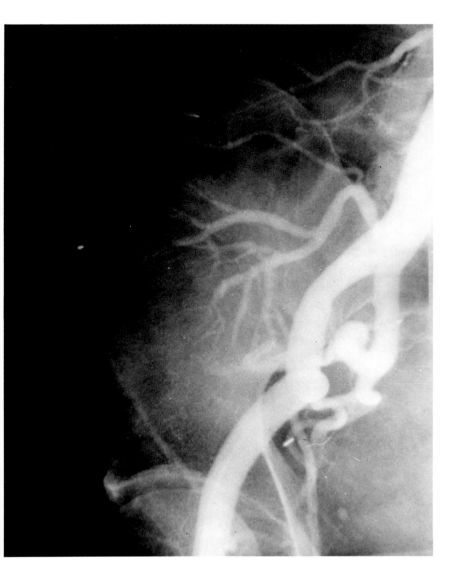

**Fig. 264.** Acute rejection (second-set type) in a sensitised patient. The early phase is marked by intense engorgement of arterioles and capillaries (MSB x 330)

**Fig. 265.** Acute second-set rejection after 7 days' transplantation. The kidney shows a swollen oedematous cortex and a dark congested medulla

**Fig. 266.** Section from specimen shown in Fig. 265 confirms the intense congestion of intertubular medullary vessels (H and E x 330)

**Fig. 267.** In acute (second-set type) rejection there is a limited cellular response, but damage to arteries (mainly as fibrinoid necrosis or thrombosis) is prominent (MSB x 198)

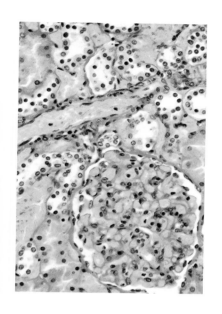

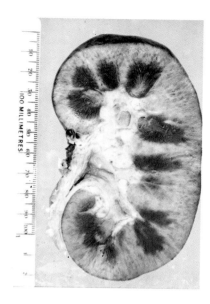

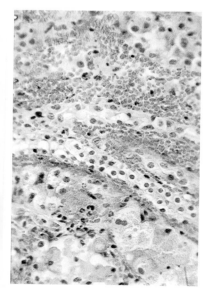

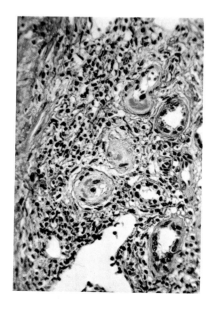

# Renal Biopsy and its Applications

PERCUTANEOUS biopsy of the kidney is now an established method of renal investigation whereby small cores of fresh renal tissue may be studied by light and electron microscopy, immunofluorescence, enzyme histochemistry or for bacterial or viral content. As a result, diagnostic accuracy is increased, the evolution of renal diseases can be followed, and structural change correlated with clinical features. The limitations of renal biopsy are imposed by sampling error on account of the small amount of tissue obtained, and by the structural composition of the tissue which may occasionally be devoid of glomeruli. The main risk to the patient is from renal bleeding, but careful selection and preparation of patients and appropriate clinical expertise can reduce this to an insignificant incidence.

Patients most profitably investigated by this technique include those with proteinuria, the nephrotic syndrome, abnormal renal function from unknown cause, or who have evidence of a "collagen disorder", renal inflammation or infection. Patients with severe hypertension, a coagulation disorder or who are unduly apprehensive should not be submitted to this investigation.

## Biopsy technique and treatment of specimens (See Appendix)

The technical methods for both these disciplines vary from one centre to another. Those outlined in the Appendix currently apply in the clinical and pathology departments participating in the renal service at the Manchester Royal Infirmary.

Figures 270–285 in the following section relate to application of renal biopsy technique. Outlines of case histories of patients from whom these illustrations were taken are given on pages 237–238.

**Fig. 268.** Taking a renal biopsy specimen. The patient lies prone; firm pillows below abdomen reduce renal movement whilst the operator introduces the biopsy needle. The kidney outline and the position of the needle are monitored (through an overhead X-ray machine) on the television screen in the background

**Fig. 269.** Component parts of the Franklin modified biopsy needle include:
  (i) needle or stylet (*above*)
  (ii) needle cover or canula (*centre*)
  (iii) toothed core prongs (*below*)
During operation, the stylet and canula are advanced to the renal cortex. The stylet is then withdrawn, replaced by the needle prongs which are then sharply pushed into the kidney cortex. Advancement of the canula now severs the renal core, which is retained by the toothed prongs during withdrawal

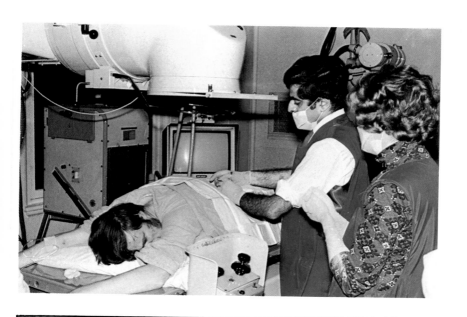

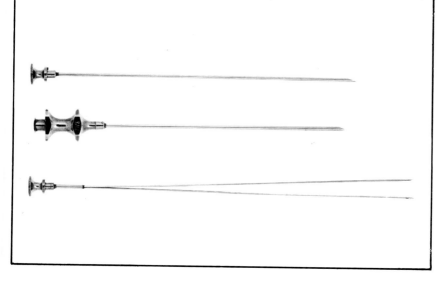

**Fig. 270.** Case 1. Renal biopsy (1961) showing a focal proliferative glomerulonephritis (PAS x 330)

**Fig. 271.** Case 1. Kidneys at autopsy (1970) showing contraction of both organs, coarse subcapsular scarring (*upper specimen*) and increased peri-pelvic fat (*lower specimen*)

**Fig. 272.** Case 1. Histology of specimens in Fig. 271 confirms widespread nephron damage—the appearances are those of a slowly progressive proliferative glomerulonephritis (PAS x 66)

**Fig. 273.** Case 1. Higher magnification of part of Fig. 272 showing glomerular sclerosis, interstitial inflammation and tubular loss (PAS x 330)

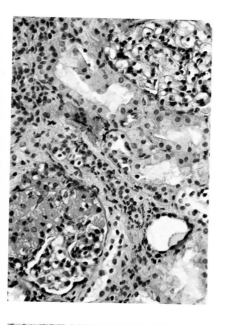

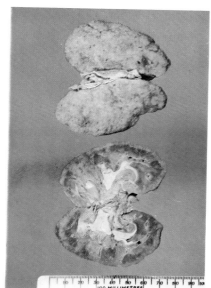

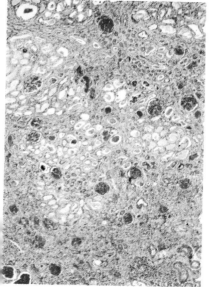

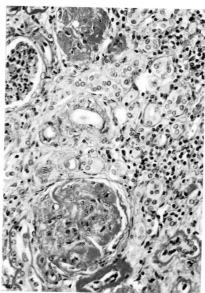

**Fig. 274.** Case 2. Renal biopsy (1969) showing proliferative changes in three glomeruli with lobulation of capillary tufts (H and E x 143)

**Fig. 275.** Case 2. Section from specimen in Fig. 276 shows the proliferative glomerular changes and fibrinoid necrosis of SLE (PAS x 330)

**Fig. 276.** Case 2. Kidneys at autopsy (1970). There is reduction of kidney size, pallor of the cortex and a fine subcapsular granularity

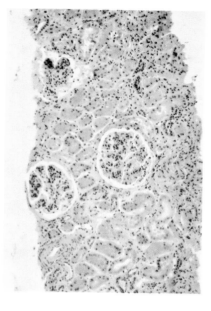

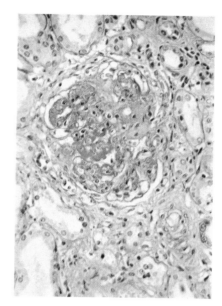

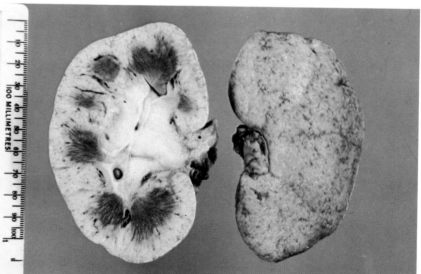

**Fig. 277.** Case 3. Renal biopsy (1968) showing uniform thickening of glomerular basement membranes in idiopathic membranous glomerulonephritis (MeS x 2080)

**Fig. 278.** Case 3. Section from kidney at autopsy (1969) showing increased basement membrane thickening and pericapsular fibrosis (H and E x 512)

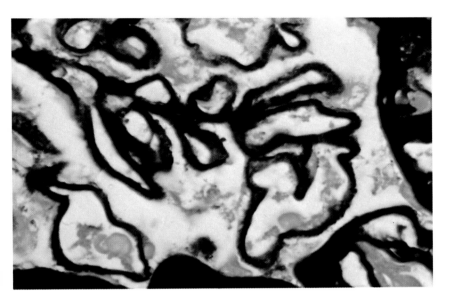

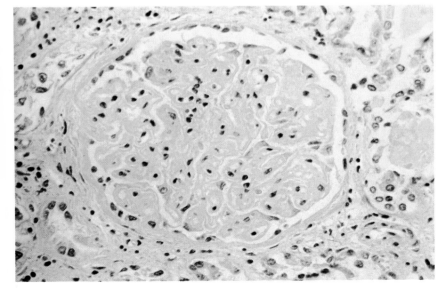

**Fig. 279.** Case 4. Renal biopsy specimen (1966) showing the proliferative changes and glomerular lobulation suggestive of SLE (H and E x 154)

**Fig. 280.** Case 4. Section from kidney at autopsy (1970) showing advanced lobular sclerosis of glomerular capillaries and secondary tubular damage (MSB x 154)

**Fig. 281.** Case 4. Different field of section (Fig. 280) showing glomerular sclerosis with fibrinoid change in glomerular capillaries and adjacent arterioles confirming severe hypertension (MSB x 480)

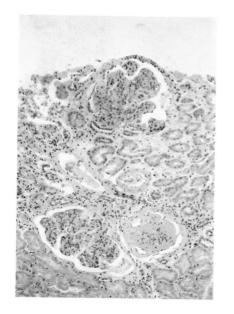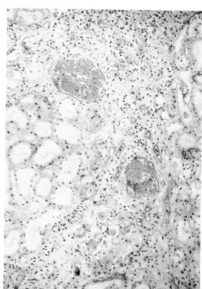
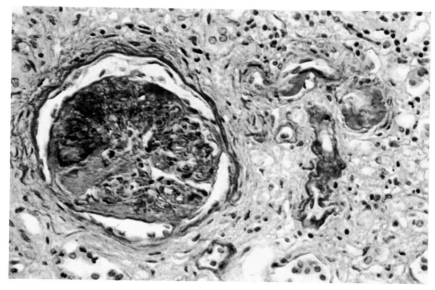

**Fig. 282.** Case 5. Renal biopsy from patient with Alport's Syndrome—a form of hereditary nephropathy—showing alternating areas of fibrosis and dilated tubules (MSB x 66)

**Fig. 283.** Case 5. Alport's Syndrome: changes of a proliferative glomerulonephritis affect some glomeruli, others appear normal (MSB x 330)

**Fig. 284.** Case 5. Alport's Syndrome. Biopsy showing focal collections of foam cells in cortex, although these are not specific to hereditary nephropathy (MSB x 330)

**Fig. 285.** Biopsy of renal transplant to investigate poor function of grafted kidney. The tubules show severe vacuolation of epithelium consistent with potassium depletion. Patient had been treated with frusemide (PAS x 550)

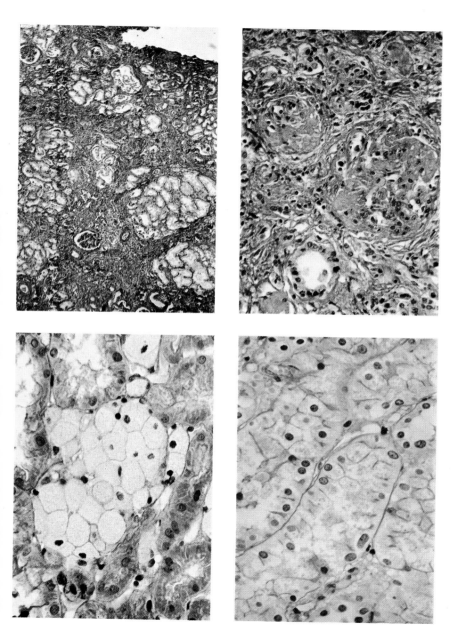

# Appendix

## Biopsy technique

The biopsies are taken from the right lower pole cortex through a Franklin modified Vim-Silverman needle after anaesthetising the skin with 3% Lignocaine and the needle track with a 1% Lignocaine solution. Intravenous 40% Hyapaque followed by an infusion of 25% Hyapaque in normal saline is used to monitor the kidney position, which is viewed on a cine-angiography x-ray machine with image intensifier. The renal core obtained is about 2 cm. long.

## Treatment of specimens

Immediately after removal, a small fragment is cut from each end of the core and fixed for electron microscopy. The remainder of the core is bisected—half being used for immunofluorescence studies and half prepared for light microscopy.

(a) *Tissue for electron microscopy:* Primary fixation in buffered 2·5% glutaraldehyde is followed by repeated washing over twenty-four hours in cacodylate buffer solution at room temperature. The tissue may then be stored in this solution at 5°C. until required for further processing. This entails post-fixation in ice-cold buffered osmium tetroxide, dehydration and embedding in Araldite or Epon. Sections of approximately 0·5 $\mu$m. thickness are stained with alkaline toluidine blue for recognition of glomeruli and tubules. Thin silver/gold sections from selected areas, mounted on grids, are double-stained with uranyl acetate lead citrate and examined electron-optically with an accelerating voltage of 60 Kv.

(b) *Tissue for immunofluorescence:* is placed on aluminium foil and rapidly frozen in an iso-pentane—solid carbon dioxide mixture. Cryostat sections of 4 $\mu$ thickness are cut and incubated in the dark at room temperature for half an hour with fluorescein-labelled, commercially-prepared anti-sera to IgA, IgG, IgM, $C_3$ fraction of complement, and fibrinogen. Sections are viewed under ultra-violet light in a darkened room. Control sections are pretreated with anti human antibody, the specificity of which can be checked at intervals by immunoelectrophoresis.

(c) *Tissue for light microscopy:* is fixed in 10% formalin/mercuric chloride solution for one hour, then dehydrated and embedded in Paraplast. Blocks are cooled in a cryostat, sections cut at $<2$ μ. thickness and stained routinely with haematoxylin/eosin (H and E), by the periodic acid-Schiff (PAS) technique, martius-scarlet-blue (MSB) and methenamine silver.

## Outline of Case Histories of Patients referred to on Pages 223–235

**Case 1.** Female; 33 years

Presented in 1958 with a complaint of nocturnal enuresis; recurrence of symptoms of mild oedema in 1961 when renal biopsy was undertaken (see Fig. 270). Subsequently improved but had further relapse in 1967 with persistent albuminuria, episodes of joint pains and skin rash. In 1970 developed signs of pericarditis with bouts of epistaxis and vomiting and increasing blood urea levels which reached 370 mg.% before death. Antinuclear factor and L.E. cells were not identified despite repeated examinations.

**Case 2.** Female; 44 years

Presented in 1964 with ankle swelling and patchy skin erythema when L.E. cells were demonstrated. Patient later developed evidence of Sjögren's syndrome (dry mouth and conjunctivae and atrophic rhinitis) and albuminuria. Renal biopsy (see Fig, 274) undertaken in 1969. Treated with steroids, diuretics and chloroquin. Final hospital admission in 1970 was on account of progressive renal failure and nephrotic syndrome.

**Case 3.** Male; 62 years

Presented in 1968 with history of long-standing pallor and puffiness; no significant antecedent history. Became progressively nephrotic; renal biopsy in September 1968 disclosed membranous glomerulonephritis (Fig. 277). Patient was re-admitted to hospital in 1969 with hypertension, failed to respond to digitalis and diuretics and died of congestive heart failure.

**Case 4.** Male; 35 years

Presented in 1966 with albuminuria. Renal biopsy disclosed a proliferative glomerulonephritis with a glomerular pattern suggestive of S.L.E. Anti-nuclear factor and S.L.E. cells were not, however, demonstrated despite repeated examinations. Under treatment, patient continued in moderate health until early 1970 when he became increasingly hypertensive and died in renal failure.

**Case 5.** Male; 43 years

Partial deafness had first been diagnosed at age of 18 months; he had suffered from "kidney trouble" from age of 7 years and his two daughters were currently subject to "kidney disease". The patient presented with eye lesions including cataract and lenticonus. He was moderately hypertensive but responded to hypotensive therapy. Renal biopsy disclosed a proliferative glomerulonephritis of rather patchy distribution (Fig. 283).

# Index